GET THE GUNK OUT

SIMPLE HEALTHY HABITS. LIFE CHANGING RESULTS.

SHANNON KADLOVSKI, BA, CNP

Copyright © 2013 **Shannon Kadlovski**
All rights reserved.
ISBN: 1482366525
ISBN 13: 9781482366525

All rights reserved. No part of this book may be reproduced in any form or by any electronic, photographic or mechanical means; nor may it be stored in a retrieval system, transmitted, or otherwise be copied for public or private use – except by a reviewer who may quote brief passages in a review or article, without permission in writing from the author.

This publication contains the opinions and ideas of its author. It is intended to provide helpful and informative material on the subjects addressed in the publication. It is sold with the understanding that the author is not engaged in rendering medical, health or any other kind of personal professional services. Nutritional and other needs vary depending on age, sex, and health status. If you suspect that you have a serious medical problem, the author strongly urges you to consult your medical, health or other competent professional for treatment.

Although the author has made every reasonable attempt to achieve complete accuracy of the content in this book, they assume no responsibility for errors or omissions. The author shall have neither liability nor responsibility to any person or entity with respect to any loss or damage caused or alleged to be caused directly or indirectly by the information, recommendations or recipes covered in this book.

Also, you should use this information as you see fit, and at your own risk. Your particular situation may not be exactly suited to the examples illustrated, and you should adjust your use of the information and recommendations accordingly.

Any trademarks, service marks, product names or named features are assumed to be the property of their respective owners, and are used only for reference. There is no implied endorsement.

Cover photo taken by TNY Photography.

www.shannonkadlovski.com

PRAISE FOR GET THE GUNK OUT

"There is truly something here for everyone looking to achieve optimal health. If you want to ease into a healthy lifestyle without feeling overwhelmed and confused, turn the page."

– *Bryce Wylde, BSc, DHMHS, Alternative Health Expert, Author of Wylde on Health*

"Shannon is my go-to when it comes to nutrition. The advice in this book changed my life. I wanted a lifestyle change and a gentle cleanse that would fit into my lifestyle and that's exactly what it did. I followed the 21-Day Gunk-Free Guide, and once the twenty-one days were complete, I continued to incorporate many of the healthy habits from this book into my daily routine. It's now just a part of my life."

– *Brianne Thom, Producer and Host - Rogers TV*

"GTGO is filled with excellent, easy to follow tips on how to clean up your lifestyle -- from what you eat, to the products you use to clean your house. Shannon's D-I-Y recipes are simple and an added bonus. I highly recommend this book for anyone looking to unjunk their lives."

– *Andrea Donsky, Founder of NaturallySavvy.com and author of "Unjunk Your Junk Food" and "Label Lessons"*

"What I love about *"Get the Gunk Out"* is its accessibility. This lifestyle – not diet – allows you to make realistic goals without feeling guilty. Using the facts, tips and recipes in this book, I am able to make smart lifestyle choices that work for me."

– *Julia Suppa, Television Host & Producer - Rogers TV*

"Shannon's practical guide for living gunk-free is the next revolution in health! It's not about deprivation; it's not a fad diet, but a true lifestyle change that will leave you feeling fabulous."

– *Emily Sawyer, Holistic Nutritionist*

"Get the Gunk Out is a practical and easy-to-follow guide to living your best life. It teaches you how to maintain a healthy lifestyle long-term, and it's not about the quick fix. I highly recommend this book to anyone who wants to look and feel great.

– Jules Lieff, Founder of Fit Organix Inc.

"Shannon's message of healthy living is very positive, and kudos to her for providing non-judgmental advice. This book will easily guide you towards a happier and healthier YOU!"

– Sarah Brager, Co-Founder of Gravitate Studio

*"Take care of your body,
it's the only place you have to live"
– Jim Rohn*

What is "Get the Gunk Out" All About?

It's about getting healthy on your own terms.

It's about incorporating simple healthy habits into your daily routine that are sustainable and maintainable long-term.

It's about being healthy and feeling great even with a busy, hectic lifestyle.

It's about learning which foods should be included and avoided as part of a gunk-free diet.

It's about not giving up the foods you love, but rather choosing healthier versions of them. (Yes, that's right, you can still eat chocolate cupcakes and be healthy).

It's about achieving your health goals without feeling like it's hard work – it's not about counting calories, fasting on juice, or taking pills and potions that are "guaranteed" to make you feel better.

It's about improving digestion, increasing energy, reducing stress, boosting immunity, reducing inflammation, and shedding unwanted pounds.

It's about making better choices when it comes to your health and nutrition.

It's about learning how to ease into a healthy lifestyle without feeling overwhelmed and confused.

It's not about being perfect or drastically changing your whole life in one day. It's about slowly introducing healthier habits into your life - **Simple healthy habits that produce life-changing results.**

It's not a diet. It's not a chore. It's simply a way of life.

Is "Get the Gunk Out" Right For Me?

You picked up this book for a reason. You're ready to make a change. You're ready to get healthy (or healthier), and *Get the Gunk Out* is going to help you do just that. Whether you currently follow a healthy diet, or have bags of fast food wrappers trapped under the front seat of your car, this book will provide you with essential tools to living a happy, healthy, gunk-free life.

Consuming processed foods, coffee, alcohol, refined sugar, and other not-so-good-for-you foods, can lead to toxic build up in our bodies. The air we breathe, the products we use in our homes, as well as our beauty care regime, can also contribute to toxic buildup and subsequent side effects. These include, bloating, heartburn, headaches, weight gain (or the inability to lose weight), acne, fatigue, anxiety, difficulty sleeping, and a host of other symptoms. *Get the Gunk Out* changes all of that. It enables you to reset your health in order to feel fabulous.

Get the Gunk Out accommodates all lifestyles and dietary habits/restrictions. It's for omnivores, vegans, vegetarians, clean eaters, fast food frequenters, those who are nut-free, gluten-free, dairy-free, and those suffering from food allergies. It's for the stay-at-home mom, the teacher, the shift worker, the office worker, the student, and everyone in between.

Get the Gunk Out is extremely beneficial for anyone suffering from high blood pressure, high cholesterol, obesity, diabetes, inflammatory conditions such as IBD and arthritis, fatigue, anxiety, lack of energy, or anyone who simply wants to live gunk-free.

Get the Gunk Out is for anyone who wants to eat better, look better, and ultimately feel better. This book is for YOU!

12 WAYS *GET THE GUNK OUT* CAN CHANGE YOUR LIFE

- Decreased gas and bloating, decreased heartburn and abdominal pain, and proper bowel movements
- Improved immune function
- Increased energy
- Improved mood
- Weight loss
- Clearer skin
- Better sleep
- Reduced stress and anxiety
- Headache relief
- Decreased cholesterol
- Reduced inflammation
- Disease prevention and improved overall health and well-being

Contents

Preface xv

Foreword xix

Introduction xxiii

LIVING GUNK-FREE 1

GUNK-FREE MENUS AND MEAL OPTIONS 10

THE GUNK-FREE DIET GUIDELINES 15

21 SIMPLE GUNK-FREE HABITS 23

    Gunk-Free Habit #1 – Set goals and go after them 23

    Gunk-Free Habit #2 – Cut the coffee and cola and sip on some tea 26

    Gunk-Free Habit #3 – Lose the booze 35

    Gunk-Free Habit #4 – Replace refined sugar 37

    Gunk-Free Habit #5 – Get more whole grains 44

    Gunk-Free Habit #6 – No more moo - 57

    Gunk-Free Habit #7 – Make fat your friend 66

    Gunk-Free Habit #8 – Eat clean pro-tein 74

    Gunk-Free Habit #9 – Time to veg 80

    Gunk-Free Habit #10 – Water, water and more water 88

    Gunk-Free Habit #11 – Squeeze some lemon 92

    Gunk-Free Habit #12 – Choose box-free Juice 96

    Gunk-Free Habit #13 – Say yes to superfoods 101

    Gunk-Free Habit #14 – Get that body moving 112

    Gunk-Free Habit #15 – Sip on a smoothie 116

    Gunk-Free Habit #16 – Make friends with probiotics 121

    Gunk-Free Habit #17 – Spice up your life 126

    Gunk-Free Habit #18 – Brush your skin, dry 131

    Gunk-Free Habit #19 – Undress your stress 133

Gunk-Free Habit #20 –
De-gunk your beauty care and household cleaners............................142

Gunk-Free Habit #21 – Clean out the clutter..150

THE 21-DAY GUNK-FREE GUIDE..**153**

GET THE GUNK OUT "CHECK IT OFF LISTS"...**167**

SIMPLE AND DELICIOUS GUNK-FREE RECIPES......................................**175**

THE GUNK-FREE DIET GROCERY LIST... **211**

ACKNOWLEDGEMENTS..**223**

RESOURCES..**225**

REFERENCES...**229**

INDEX...**235**

Recipe Index

For additional recipes and gunk-free meal ideas see page 10

Breakfast
Whole grain French toast – 177
Gluten-free pancakes – 178
Morning Muesli – 178

Soups
Butternut squash soup – 201
Split pea soup – 202
Broccoli and cauliflower soup – 203

Salads/Sides
Sesame and garlic spinach – 85
Kale and cabbage coleslaw – 86
Apple, beet and sweet potato quinoa salad – 195
Roasted beets – 196
Sweet potato salad – 197
Whole grain pasta salad – 198
Edamame and avocado salad – 199
Tempeh and quinoa salad – 193

Mains
Hearty turkey chili – 187
Tasty tamari tempeh – 188
Quinoa veggie burgers – 189
Baked chicken (or turkey) meatballs – 190
Tempeh lettuce wraps – 191
Maple miso glazed salmon – 192

Juices and Tea
Green juice – 85
Refreshingly soothing lemonade – 93
Lemon and apple cider vinegar detox drink – 94
Clean and green juice – 98
Digestive juice – 98
Love your liver juice – 99
V-7 juice – 99
Sweet beet juice – 99
Parsley and ginger tea – 130

Smoothies
Heavenly chocolate protein smoothie – 180
Scrumptious superfood smoothie – 180
The Energizer Smoothie – 181
Pumpkin Spice Smoothie – 181
Coco-Nutty Smoothie - 182

Dips/Spreads
Hearty hummus – 182
Avocado and goat cheese dip – 183
Simple salsa – 184
Creamy chocolate hazelnut spread – 186
Raspberry chia jam – 103
Dairy-free cheese – 64

Sauces/Dressings
Oil and vinegar dressing – 198
Basil pesto dressing – 199
Creamy avocado dressing – 199
Zesty lemon dressing – 93
Pineapple sauce – 184
Garlic parsley sauce – 185

Snacks and Desserts
Kale chips – 84
Chocolate chia pudding – 102
Scrumptious honey sesame crackers – 204
Chocolate avocado pudding – 205
Date squares – 206
Chocolate squash brownies – 207
Chewy chocolate granola bars – 208
Zucchini banana loaf – 209
Ice no-cream – 63

Beauty and Household Care
Homemade body lotion, facemasks, and hair care – 145
Homemade household cleaners – 148

Other
Chia gel – 102

Preface

> "A year from now, you will wish you had started today"
> – Karen Lamb

I wasn't always into healthy living and wholesome eating. In fact, I spent the better part of my teens and early twenties living on fast food, frozen dinners, and any candy or chocolate that I could get my hands on. I never really thought about the foods that I was eating or what they might be doing to my health – I just ate to eat.

I was surrounded by family illness, from Crohn's disease, to colitis, and cancer, and in my early twenties I became extremely ill – constantly anxious, always exhausted, unable to focus or barely function. I spent days in bed, paralyzed by fear, hoping that when I woke up, my living nightmare would be over. My drug of choice at the time was food. I ate everything and anything, and as a result, developed severe acid reflux and irritable bowel syndrome. Of course, I gained almost forty pounds, which didn't help with my physical state (or emotional state, for that matter). It was a vicious cycle that seemed like it would never end.

I remember driving down highway 401 in Toronto one day, when out of nowhere, I felt as though I couldn't breathe. My heart began to race and my throat felt like it was about to close. I began sweating, and the world felt like it was spinning around me. I looked into the rearview mirror at myself, noticing that my face was completely white. I knew at that moment that I was either going to faint, or die. I quickly pulled off to the side of the road and stuck my head between my knees. I cried.

I had had enough. Somehow, I managed to call 911. After three hours in the hospital, I was sent home with an anti-anxiety pill and advice from the doctor to "just try to relax".

I saw one doctor after the next, had dozens of tests done, and after each visit was told that it was "just stress" and it was "all in my head". I was then handed a series of prescriptions for anti-anxiety meds. I never filled them.

My stomach pains got worse and worse, and again, doctor after doctor simply handed me prescription antacids. I took them. I was desperate. But, even after weeks of antacid treatment, I was still in serious pain. I went through cycles of eating everything in sight, to not being able to eat anything at all. I knew my body and I knew myself, and what I knew more than anything, was that it was something bigger than being "just in my head". Yes, granted, I was stressed and dealing with a lot at the time, but I knew there was something more to it. I knew that this wasn't my typical day-to-day stress, but that something seriously wrong was happening inside of me. I didn't want to spend the rest of my life taking medication that would merely mask my symptoms, rather than deal with the root of what was really going on.

After spending countless hours sitting on the floor in the middle of my local bookstore (with a sugar-filled coffee in hand – it was the only way that I could get through the day), devouring as many health and wellness books as I could, I discovered that my chronic fatigue, frequent panic attacks, and dizziness were all a result of extreme adrenal fatigue. In other words, the systems in my body that regulate my nervous system were way out of whack and not functioning at their highest potential. But, why and how was this happening?

I continued reading, and then read some more, and what I discovered was that my lifestyle habits and incredibly poor diet were directly affecting the way my adrenal system was functioning (or not functioning). My incredibly poor diet, made up of coffee, soda, bagels, fast food burgers, sugar-filled chocolate, and white pasta with tomato sauce, was not only contributing to my weight gain, but was also the leading cause of my severe acid reflux and anxiety.

I made the choice to rid my diet of refined sugar, processed foods, and excessive amounts of red meat. I began eating healthier foods, drinking lemon water daily, practicing yoga, and really tuning in to my body in order to improve the quality of my health. Within two months, I felt more alive, more vibrant and healthier than ever before – not to mention, I had lost almost twenty pounds. My digestion not only improved, but it was impeccable. I worked to support my body and my adrenal system with the proper care it deserved, and I learned how to cope with my stress. I practiced proper breathing and relaxation techniques, and eventually mastered overcoming panic attacks without any kind of medication.

My path was then clear; I had to help others.

After receiving my Bachelor's degree from York University, I took my passion to the Institute of Holistic Nutrition, where I graduated with first class honors and obtained my Certified Nutritional Practitioner (CNP) designation. I made it my mission to educate and help as many people as I could about the amazing, life-changing benefits that proper diet and healthy habits can have on our lives.

> *"Making small, realistic changes to your diet and lifestyle can have a powerful, positive impact on the quality of your life".*

My approach to health is simple – eat wholesome, natural, clean foods as much as possible and try to minimize the amount of processing and chemicals involved. Don't give up the foods you love, just choose healthier versions of them. Don't take yourself too seriously or be too hard on yourself, it's all about balance. Take the time everyday to focus on you – breathe and de-stress. Never "go on a diet", but instead commit to making healthier diet and lifestyle choices that work for you.

When it comes to healing from illness, instead of simply masking symptoms with "band- aid" medications, work to treat the root cause of your symptoms from the inside out. Fill your body with vitamins, minerals and other essential nutrients that will support you on your path to wellness.

So, now it's up to you. Take this book and allow it to help you make the changes that you need to live the life you want to live. Live healthy, live happy, live gunk-free.

Foreword

By Bryce Wylde, Alternative Health Expert. BSc, DHMHS

The search for a single pathogen — a single external agent — as the cause of a particular disease is not a complete solution. Our health appears rather to be the end result of many cumulative factors that go beyond even our genes and our environment.

My experience with my patients has brought home to me that human health consists of an interplay of variables that include our genetics, our environment, our toxic load, our stress accumulation, our nutrition and emotional state, our exposure to microbes, our level of fitness, and a plethora of other factors. For most, that doesn't precipitate any new epiphany. Each of us has a certain and very individual ability to manage these factors. The limit of that unique ability - the point at which, if we exceed it, our health fails - is our individual health threshold.

If we imagine a thermometer that registers the sum of all these interacting factors, our health threshold is the boiling point. By analogy then, like water, think of your individual health threshold as 100 degrees Celsius. The capacity for managing the various influences that affect our health is different for each of us because for some, stress, for example, accounts for 20 degrees, where for others, stress may account for 50 degrees at any given time. For some, poor diet may account for 30 degrees, but for others, it could be 70 degrees due to a genetic predisposition toward obesity. Nonetheless, when we are pushed past our individual thresholds, we are no more able to remain healthy than water can prevent itself from boiling when it's heated to the boiling point. Today, many of us run so dangerously close to that threshold that we increase our probability of an early decline in the functioning of our bodies. For time immemorial humans have been exposed to microbes, stress, malnutrition, and extremely harsh conditions. But today, the "gunk" we're exposed to is hands down the biggest contributing factor that pushes us past our human health threshold - often to our breaking point.

We may be living longer than the generations who came before us, but we are living longer with chronic disease and discomfort. We are "gunked up." Our health "temperature" constantly rises with our increasing levels of stress, environmental burdens, and in particular our exposure to the "gunk" in our diet and environment, just as the mercury in a thermometer slides up in response to an increase in temperature.

Since the Second World War, an estimated 85,000 synthetic chemicals have been registered in North America (many more are unregistered!). Often these chemicals are found in our food and water supply or end up in us unwittingly. How do we lessen the burden on our individual health threshold? Shannon Kadlovski has a simple and effective plan to help. How about avoiding the "gunk" in the first place!

Shannon is a visionary proponent of nutrition, charismatic media personality, astute entrepreneur, sound nutritionist, and healthy lifestyle specialist.

Throughout "Get the Gunk Out", Shannon shares key tips on living Gunk-Free" and offers "how to" advice on turning healthy into a habit. Along the way "Get the Gunk Out" provides concise action plans, check lists, 21-day gunk free detox, and grocery lists for healthier, optimal living through diet and lifestyle. Plus, Kadlovski packs the book with all natural, healthy, and delicious recipes that help you stick the course. From diet and digestive health - and an approach to achieving optimal digestion - to recommendations on how to set realistic goals and methods to de-stress, to skin brushing and beauty care, there is truly something here for everyone looking to achieve optimal health.

Can we really have our cake, eat it, AND be healthy too? Yes, so long as you first get the gunk out! In this manual packed with small, realistic modifications, Nutritionist Shannon Kadlovski shows you how your diet and lifestyle can have a powerful impact on the quality of your life.

If you want to ease into a healthy lifestyle without feeling overwhelmed and confused, turn the page.

Bryce Wylde, Alternative Health Expert. BSc, DHMHS
Author of Wylde On Health
CEO, Wylde About Health Inc.

Introduction

Gunk

- Food that is processed, refined and simply unhealthy.
- Dietary and lifestyle habits that contribute to illness and unpleasant symptoms.
- Toxic build up in the body from unhealthy food, environmental toxins, toxins in beauty care products and household cleaners.
- Recurring physical and emotional stress.
- Anything that prevents you from living a healthy, nourished life.

GET THE GUNK OUT. GET THE GOOD STUFF IN. IT'S AS SIMPLE AS THAT!

Congratulations on taking the first step towards becoming a healthier, gunk-free *you*! With this book, you will learn simple, realistic, and effective ways to eat better, look better, and ultimately feel better. Whether you plan to follow the twenty-one day gunk-free guide (page 153), or choose to use this book as a guide to changing your diet and lifestyle habits over a longer period of time, *Get the Gunk Out* will enable you to achieve your goals.

Think of this book as a healthy diet and lifestyle transformation guide. This is not a fad diet or strict and complicated diet plan. It doesn't require counting calories or grams of fat, and certainly does not place you into a specific category or group based on your age, weight and height. This book is about learning what works for you, as an individual.

This book will teach you how to make simple, step-by-step changes that slowly ease you into a healthier lifestyle. It does not require you to follow a perfect diet all of the time, but rather teaches you simple healthy habits that can be incorporated into your daily routine without feeling overwhelmed.

This book enables you to make choices. It provides you with the tools you need to make healthy changes, but allows you to slowly introduce them into your life, at your own pace. It enables you to pick and choose from the gunk-free habits outlined in this book as you see fit. So, whether your goal is to simply eat more vegetables, learn how to include more fiber in your diet, decrease gas and bloating, get better sleep, or do a complete diet and lifestyle overhaul, this book makes it easy for you to do just that.

How This Book Works

With this book, you will learn how to follow a gunk-free diet, as well as simple healthy habits that work to improve digestion, promote detoxification, decrease inflammation, increase energy, promote weight loss, and lead to overall better health and vitality. These are simple, realistic habits, that when slowly incorporated into your life, will enable you to feel your best. The idea is not to make all of these healthy changes in one day, but to slowly introduce them into your life, day-by-day (or week-by-week, month-by-month, depending on your lifestyle).

You may choose to incorporate one or two gunk-free habits into your life on a daily basis, or make bigger changes by incorporating all twenty-one. You may choose to incorporate the healthy habits in the order that they appear, or pick and choose from them as you see fit.

The idea is to at least try all of the healthy habits at some point. Some suggestions may work for you, while others may not. We are all different, so what works for one person may not work for another. There is nothing wrong with this, and in fact, that is what this book is all about – finding out what works for *you*.

Twenty-One is The Magic Number

It takes twenty-one days to make or break a habit, and it also takes twenty-one days for our taste buds to adapt to new tastes. Twenty-one days is the ideal amount of time necessary to reset your diet and your health. The twenty-one day gunk-free guide (page 153) enables you to apply the habits outlined in this book in a slow and steady manner, giving your body and mind time to adapt to the changes taking place.

Whether you choose to follow the twenty-one day gunk-free guide or not, you will notice that there are suggestions throughout the book that recommend trying particular habits for any consecutive twenty-one day period. After that time, you will reassess how you feel, and decide whether or not that particular gunk-free habit is something that you want to live with long-term.

Living Gunk-Free

Gunk-free living is about eliminating all of the things that weigh you down and prevent you from feeling your best. It's about removing the gunk from your diet, removing the gunk from your body, and removing the excess gunk from your life. Cutting out the bad stuff is important, but it's just as important to make sure to include the good stuff. Living gunk-free is about incorporating simple diet and lifestyle habits into your life that help to reset your health and leave you feeling better than ever.

Living gunk-free is simple - follow the gunk-free diet (page 15) and practice some of the simple gunk-free habits outlined in this book.

LIVING GUNK-FREE 101

Making healthy changes can be overwhelming when you are uncertain about what to buy at the grocery store, what to look for and avoid on product labels, how much of certain foods to eat, what to eat when dining out, how to eat healthy on-the-go, how to plan meals, and how to decipher misleading marketing on product labels.

Once you are equipped with the necessary tools to master all of the confusion, living gunk-free is a breeze.

UNDERSTANDING PRODUCT LABELS

Often we look directly at the nutrition facts (calories, fat, carbs) before ever reading the actual ingredients. And, although the nutrition facts are important (like making sure the product does not contain saturated or trans fats, and is high in fiber and low in sodium), it is important to first examine where these nutrients are coming from and the *types* of ingredients that are in these products.

It is important to choose products made with mostly natural, wholesome ingredients, such as whole grains, nuts, seeds, healthy oils (such as olive, sesame, and coconut oils), as well as natural sweeteners (such as honey, coconut sugar, molasses, and date syrup). Words such as polyunsaturated, monounsaturated, raw, sprouted, and whole, indicate that the item is likely a healthy and nutritious choice.

If the list of ingredients in overwhelmingly long and contains words that are tricky to pronounce, simply put it down and move on to the next – this indicates that (most likely) the product contains synthetic, unhealthy ingredients.

We want to choose products that do NOT contain the following words:

- Hydrogenated
- Partially hydrogenated
- Trans fat
- Fructose
- Sucrose
- Dextrose
- Glucose
- Corn syrup
- High fructose corn syrup
- Sucralose
- Aspartame
- Saccharine
- Acesulfame
- Sodium nitrate
- Sodium sulfite
- Sodium propionate
- Artificial colorings
- Monosodium Glutamate (MSG) and other names for it such as:
    » Textured protein
    » Autolyzed yeast
    » Yeast extract

- Yeast food
- Glutamate or Glutamic Acid
- Autolyzed plant protein
- Sodium caseinate
- Calcium caseinate
- Hydrolyzed protein
- Hydrolyzed vegetable protein(HVP)
- Hydrolyzed plant protein (HPP)
- Soy protein extract

- Artificial flavors
- Maltodextrin
- Polydextrose
- Phosphoric acid
- White or refined flour
- Anything with a number – for example, blue #2, blue #1, yellow #6

HOW TO OUTSMART MISLEADING MARKETING ON FOOD LABELS

1. Buy mostly fresh, organic foods

Stock your cart with **fresh fruits and veggies** (lots of different colors), **whole grains** (brown rice, quinoa, oats, etc.), **nuts and seeds** – and butters made from these (almonds, walnuts, flaxseeds, chia seeds, hemp seeds, etc...) **fresh, lean meats** - chicken, fish, turkey, etc., and **legumes** (chickpeas, kidney beans, lima beans, etc.).

* Buying fresh, whole foods eliminates the guesswork, as these items do not come with fancy labels and marketing slogans. They are good, clean foods that our bodies need to stay healthy.

2. Be careful of products that are marketed as low-fat, non-fat, and "only 100-calories"

The truth is, that although these items may appear to be less fattening, they actually contribute to more hunger and weight gain. When the fat is removed from items such as milk or yogurt for example, they replace the lost fat with added sugar. Added sugar contributes to the overproduction of insulin, which leads to fat storage. The added sugar also makes us feel hungrier and sends us back to the kitchen for more snack foods.

Have you ever really looked at the ingredients in those 100-calorie snack packs? The list of ingredients is quite scary. If an item is only 100-calories, that means that we will eat less and lose weight, right? Wrong! In fact, the exact opposite is true. These 100-calorie snacks are loaded with refined sugar, added fats (the "bad" fats), tons of added sodium, and a long list of other chemicals that are barely pronounceable.

What does that mean? It means that instead of containing items that will actually help to satisfy our cravings, and provide us with sustained energy, they contain artificial ingredients that our bodies don't recognize, and simply don't know how to metabolize. Consuming artificial ingredients such as, **monosodium glutamate, partially hydrogenated soybean oil, and artificial color**, which are all found in many of the 100-calorie snacks, is what causes us to feel irritable, tired and bloated. They work to make us hungrier, and actually contribute to storing more calories as fat. In the long run, we end up eating more and storing more fat. Not quite what we were promised by the marketing companies.

3. Stay away from items marked "all natural" unless they are actually 100% natural

How do we tell the difference between items labeled "all natural" and items that are actually 100% natural? Simple. We look at the ingredients. If you see any of these words on your food label, you can be certain that it is **not** actually 100% natural:

* **Sugar, sucrose, sucralose, maltodextrin, artificial color or flavoring, partially hydrogenated or hydrogenated oils, high fructose corn syrup, modified corn starch and monosodium glutamate.**

Many products claim to be all-natural, but after further investigation, we realize that they contain processed and artificial ingredients. But, how can this be?

The Food and Drug Administration does not have strict guidelines for labeling products as all natural, and although manufacturers are required to list all of the ingredients in a food product, they are not required to have the rest of the information on the package reflect the actual contents.

The FDA's guidelines: *Anything derived from plants, animals or elements found on planet Earth can earn the "all natural" label.*

The problem is, that even though certain foods may originate from natural sources (like sugar, for example, which comes from sugar cane), it is the processing of these foods that is unnatural, not the source of the food itself. When you process and alter the chemical structure of foods into forms that no longer appear anywhere in nature, that food is no longer natural – regardless of where it came from originally.

The bottom line is that we want to consume mostly fresh, organic, whole foods such as, fruits, vegetables, legumes, nuts, seeds, whole grains and high quality meats. Although there are some truly good products that come in boxes, it is important to carefully examine the ingredients before ever trusting the fancy labels and marketing slogans. Remember to read your labels in order to decipher the "truly good" from the "misleading and simply wrong".

MEAL TIME – BREAKING IT DOWN

It is important to eat a balanced meal at each meal. Your plate should consist of mostly protein (lean meats, fish, poultry, tempeh - limit red meat), complex carbohydrates (sweet potatoes, legumes, whole grains), as well as roughly ten percent of your meal consisting of healthy fats (avocado, nuts, seeds, and healthy oils). In addition, always fill your plate with fresh or steamed vegetables. Unless you are advised to for medical reasons, NEVER cut out an entire food group (such as carbohydrates), as this can be very dangerous to your health.

It is important to consume three well-balanced meals each day, as well as two to three snacks (in between breakfast and lunch, in between lunch and dinner, and perhaps one more after dinner (depending on the time at which you ate dinner). Never skip breakfast – starting your day off with fuel from food is essential in order to keep blood sugar balanced and prevent our bodies from storing excess fat while it goes into starvation mode. It is important to avoid eating at least two to three hours before going to bed. Eating before bed disrupts sleep patterns and makes for restless, non-restorative sleeps.

Getting the gunk out and adopting healthier eating habits is not about limiting calories or daily food intake, but rather learning which TYPES of foods you should be eating and which TYPES you should be avoiding. When it comes to portion size, it is important not to overeat, but it is just as important to not deprive yourself if you are hungry.

Everyone's daily food intake needs are different, since after all, we are all different in terms of weight, height, activity level, etc., Because of this, it is important to take note of how you feel before, during and after each meal. Try to avoid eating simply out of boredom, but rather check in with yourself to see whether you are truly hungry. If you are hungry, eat, but eat the good stuff. If a half-cup of rice with vegetables simply doesn't hit the spot, wait twenty minutes, reassess your hunger, and eat another half-cup if you are truly still hungry. You will likely notice that eating clean wholesome foods enables you to feel more satisfied than you normally would while consuming a diet of refined foods and sugar-filled drinks.

- A typical portion of meat or fish is about 3 ounces - about the size of your fist.
- A typical portion of whole grains (pasta, rice, cereal, dry grains) is about ½ cup.
- A typical portion of legumes (beans, peas and lentils) and other complex carbohydrates (sweet potato, squash, parsnip, corn) is about ½ - ¾ cup.
- A typical portion of fruit is ½ cup or a medium sized fruit.
- A typical portion of vegetables is ½ cup and about 1 cup for leafy green vegetables.
- A typical portion of nuts and seeds is about a handful of nuts and/or seeds or 1-2 tablespoons of oil or nut/seed butter.

If you fall off track here and there, that's okay. Do not feel guilty, but rather get right back on track the next day. Again, healthy living is not about being perfect – it's about following a healthy diet as much as possible, but allowing yourself the freedom to just be human.

Healthy eating doesn't have to be difficult, and you don't have to be an experienced cook to reap the benefits. If you love to cook, great! Take some time to play around in the kitchen. Allow yourself to get creative and use new ingredients that you may not have used before. If cooking isn't really your thing, or if you are always on-the-go and simply too busy to cook, this book will teach you how to eat healthier without having to spend too much time in the kitchen. **The bottom line is that whether you use your oven to cook food, or use it as an extra storage space for your clothes, healthy eating is simple and achievable.**

If you are the don't-love-to-cook type, and you're up for the challenge, try to get yourself into the kitchen at least a few times per week. Eating healthy doesn't have to mean slaving in the kitchen for hours, and in fact, a healthy meal can be prepared in less time than it takes to drive to your local fast food restaurant and wait in the drive-through line. This book includes simple, delicious recipes that even the non-cooks can make. So, give it a try, you might impress yourself!

Try to keep your diet interesting and avoid getting stuck in a food rut, where you eat the same thing day after day. This can get boring and eventually turn you off of certain foods.

Use the gunk-free diet guidelines (page 15) as the basis for your meal choices. There is plenty of variety and many different ways to incorporate these foods into your daily meals. If you ever feel stuck on what to eat however, choose from the gunk-free meal options on page 10. These are simply suggestions, so feel free to add or remove any ingredients that you wish.

ALWAYS BE PREPARED

The best thing to do in order to be prepared for those "I don't feel like cooking" days is to pick one or two days per week to prepare some staple foods. This way, you will have healthy items on hand for those extra busy or lazy days. Store your pre-made foods in the refrigerator (depending on their shelf life) or freeze them, and defrost as needed.

- Make a large batch of steel cut oats and keep them in the fridge for three to four days. Each morning, scoop out a portion and reheat on the stovetop for a few minutes. Then, simply add in your favorite toppings (cinnamon, fruit, nuts, seeds and/or natural sweetener of choice). The same goes for quinoa, pasta, or rice.
- Pre-wash and cut fresh vegetables and keep them in airtight containers in the fridge. This way, they are all ready to be thrown into a salad or to be taken for a snack. Sometimes the thought of having to cut up all of the veggies can turn you off of wanting to eat them, so having them pre-cut and ready-to-go is a great help.
- Make a large pot of soup and freeze individual portions in the freezer. Defrost as needed in the fridge, and reheat on the stovetop.
- Make a large batch of your favourite snack recipes (page 204) and store them in an airtight container. Or, store them in the fridge or freezer depending on how quickly you are going to consume them. Having healthy snacks handy is a great way to avoid reaching for gunk-filled goodies.

WHAT TO EAT WHEN YOU'RE DINING OUT

- Load up on veggies – replace a side order of fries with healthier options (steamed or raw vegetables or side salad).
- Choose foods that are steamed or baked, as opposed to fried.
- Avoid high fat dressings (ask for oil and vinegar or dressing on the side).

- Avoid foods cooked in butter, oil, and heavy sauces - ask for these ingredients on the side, or to be cooked without.
- Stick to whole grains - order whole grain pasta or pizza (if option is available), and ask for whole grain bread instead of white.
- Order water instead of soda pop or alcohol.
- Ask for the nutrition information of your chosen meal, or check online ahead of time.

GUNK-FREE MEAL TIPS

- Always include at least one cup of fresh vegetables at each meal (leafy greens, cucumbers, peppers, carrots, tomatoes, beets, etc.) or steamed vegetables (Brussels sprouts, broccoli, asparagus or veggies of choice).
- Marinate your meat/fish/tempeh/chicken using Braggs or Tamari sauces, fresh lemon, 1-2 cloves of fresh crushed garlic, and olive oil.
- Use 1-2 tsp. of any spice to enhance flavour (can combine more than one spice in your dishes) - ginger, parsley, dill, rosemary, basil, thyme, chives, paprika, turmeric, black pepper, sea salt.

GUNK-FREE MEAL OPTIONS

Breakfast

Option 1
½ cup of plain, steel cut oatmeal or ½ cup cooked quinoa with 1 tbsp. of ground flax seeds and 1-2 tsp. of cinnamon. Can use stevia, pure maple syrup, or raw honey to sweeten. Can add sliced banana, fresh berries, and/or goji berries. Can add any milk alternative.
Option 2
2 slices of whole grain or gluten-free toast with 1-2 tbsp. natural almond butter or sunflower seed butter. Sprinkle with cinnamon and ground flax seeds or chia seeds.
Option 3
3 egg whites or 2 egg whites and 1 whole egg (cook anyway you like – scrambled, omelet, sunny side up). Use grape seed oil or ghee when cooking eggs, or use a non-stick pan. Serve with 2 slices of whole grain or gluten-free bread, and vegetables or fresh fruit.
Option 4
½ cup plain, unsweetened kefir, Greek yogurt, or coconut yogurt with 1 tbsp. goji berries, 1 tbsp. chia seeds, 1 tsp. cinnamon, ¼ cup fresh blueberries/raspberries. Add ¼ tsp. matcha green tea powder for extra energy.
Option 5
Protein smoothie – See recipes on pages 180-182.
Option 6
Gluten-free granola with almond milk (or other milk alternative). Can add fresh berries/dried coconut/raisins.
Option 7
Gluten-free pancakes topped with fresh berries or other fresh fruit, 1 tbsp. pure maple syrup, ¼ tsp. cinnamon and 1 tbsp. ground flax seeds - see recipe on page 178.

Lunch

Option 1
100% whole grain tortilla with grilled chicken, vegetables (celery, cucumber, mushrooms, lettuce, tomato, etc.), ½ an avocado – can dress with balsamic vinegar, lemon, olive oil.
Option 2
1 cup of cooked brown rice or quinoa with 1-2 cups of vegetables and 3-4 oz. grilled chicken, tempeh, beans, or salmon.
Option 3
Salad with legumes (black beans, lentils, kidney beans, navy beans, garbanzo beans), vegetables (beets, cucumber, peppers, spinach, broccoli, carrots, eggplant, etc.), ¼ cup of nuts or seeds (almonds, walnuts, pecans, sesame seeds), and cold pressed oil for dressing (flax seed oil/sesame seed oil/ olive oil), or any dressing on the gunk-free list.
Option 4
Egg and avocado sandwich: 2 pieces gluten-free bread with 1 hard-boiled egg (chopped), and ¼ avocado. Add tomatoes, cucumber, lettuce, and onions. * Can use marinated tempeh (page 188) in place of egg.
Option 5
Hummus and avocado sandwich: 2 pieces gluten-free bread with 2 tbsp. hummus and ¼ avocado. Add tomatoes, cucumber, lettuce, and onions.
Option 6
1 cup apple, beet and sweet potato quinoa salad (page 195).
Option 7
1 cup of split pea soup with ½ sandwich (see options 4 and 5) or create your own sandwich on whole grain bread.

Dinner

Option 1
1 cup of brown rice or 1 cup of quinoa. Add lightly steamed vegetables and 3-4 oz. grilled chicken or ½ cup of sprouted tofu or tempeh. Can use Braggs or Tamari sauce.
Option 2
1 cup whole grain pasta with mixed vegetables. Add chicken or fish. Can also use ground turkey or chicken in a homemade tomato sauce.
Option 3
3-4 oz of grilled chicken or salmon, 1 sweet potato (can season with 1 tbsp of olive oil and 1 tsp of cinnamon), and fresh or steamed vegetables.
Option 4
1 cup butternut squash soup. 3-4 oz of chicken or fish with a side salad or mixed steamed vegetables.
Option 5
1-2 cups hearty turkey chili (page 187).
Option 6
1 quinoa veggie burger (page 189) and 1/2 cup edamame and avocado salad (page 199).
Option 7
1 cup split pea soup (page 202) with ½ sandwich (see lunch options 4 and 5) or create your own sandwich on whole grain bread. 1 cup fresh or steamed vegetables.

GUNK-FREE SNACKS

- Fresh vegetables (celery, carrots, cucumber, pepper) with 2 tbsp. hummus (page 182) or avocado and goat cheese dip (page 183).
- ½ cup plain, unsweetened kefir, Greek Yogurt, or coconut yogurt, with 2 tbsp. of ground flax seeds, 1 tsp. cinnamon and a handful of raw nuts and/or fresh fruit.
- 1 medium sized fruit with 1-2 tbsp. of sunflower seed butter, almond butter, or any other nut/seed butter.
- ¼ - ½ cup of trail mix (mixed nuts, seeds, and dried fruit).
- ½ cup simple salsa (page 184) with honey sesame crackers (page 204).
- 2 hard-boiled eggs with fresh vegetables (carrots and celery).
- Protein smoothie (pages 180-182).
- Air popped, non-GMO popcorn.
- Any of the homemade snack recipes (page 204).

The Gunk-Free Diet Guidelines

The gunk-free diet is in fact not a diet at all, but rather a dietary guideline based on incorporating wholesome, natural, clean foods into your diet, while limiting/eliminating those that are heavily processed, refined, and unhealthy. It's about eating foods from the "gunk-free" section and avoiding foods from the "gunk-filled" section. It's simple. **You don't have to worry about counting calories, grams of fat, or measuring out exact serving sizes. The gunk-free diet is about focusing on the *types* of foods that you are eating, rather than the amount.**

The gunk-free diet is about eliminating the stress and confusion that is often associated with "dieting". It's about adopting habits that help to make healthy eating simple, realistic, and maintainable.

Gunk-free eating is about eliminating the foods and lifestyle habits that contribute to poor health. But more importantly, it's about consuming more of the foods and practicing more of the lifestyle habits that help to promote good health.

Incorporating the gunk-free diet into your life is not something that should be accomplished in one day. **The goal** is to eventually eat from the "gunk-free" list and completely avoid the "gunk-filled" list long-term. Taking baby steps, and slowly changing the *way* you eat and the *types* of foods you eat, is the way to go. **Don't think of this as a diet, but rather a healthy lifestyle change, accomplished over time.**

"Be not afraid of going slowly; be afraid only of standing still"
– Chinese proverb

GUNK-FREE FOODS TO EAT

For a complete grocery list, including suggested brands, see page 211.

Protein

Protein powder

Vegan protein (no additives or artificial/refined sweeteners), 100% New Zealand whey protein isolate/concentrate (no additives or artificial/refined sweeteners)

Legumes

Chickpeas, kidney beans, lentils, navy beans, peas, pinto beans, red lentils, black beans, adzuki beans, mixed beans, split peas, mung beans, soybeans (edamame – frozen), tofu (sprouted), tempeh

Fish – wild caught when possible

Salmon, mackerel, halibut, tuna, cod, haddock, sardines, snapper, tuna, trout, tilapia

Poultry – lean, free-range & organic when possible

Chicken and turkey (fresh or ground – not processed), quail, duck

Red Meat – lean, grass-fed & organic when possible (consume red meat in moderation).

Beef, lamb, venison, veal

Eggs - free-run

Nuts and seeds - raw, unsalted

Almonds, cashews, Brazil nuts, walnuts, macadamia nuts, pecans, sesame seeds, sunflower seeds, pumpkin seeds, flax seeds, hemp seeds, chia seeds

Nut and seed butters - organic when possible, free of refined sugar

Nut butters, sunflower seed butter, pumpkin seed butter, tahini, organic peanut butter (avoid non-organic peanut butter)

Carbohydrates

Hot Cereals

Oatmeal (plain steel cut oats or rolled oats) – avoid instant oatmeal with added flavours/sugar. Opt for gluten-free oats when possible, quinoa and/or quinoa flakes (raw grains to be cooked), oat bran

Dry Cereals

100% whole grain cereal without added sugar, quinoa puffs, brown rice cereal, granola (without added sugar)

Whole grains/Pasta/Rice/Flour/Crackers/Bread/Cookies/Snacks

Quinoa, buckwheat, spelt, rye, brown rice and brown rice pasta, millet, barley, kamut, corn, teff, amaranth, brown rice crackers, 100% whole grain crackers, plain rice cakes, cookies and snacks made with whole grains, no added sugar, color or artificial ingredients. (Those with gluten sensitivities should avoid spelt, rye, wheat, and oats.)

Fruits & Vegetables

Any and all fruits and vegetables are acceptable, except those that cause a reaction. Avoid grapefruit if on medication. *See pages 82-83 for detailed list of fruits and vegetables.*

Vegetables – organic when possible

Collard greens, kale, spinach, broccoli, cauliflower, bok choy, carrots, celery, beets, tomato, cucumber, bell peppers, eggplant, mushrooms, sweet potato, butternut squash, asparagus, zucchini, other fresh vegetables, frozen vegetables.

Fruits – organic when possible (fresh or frozen)

Avocado, blueberries, blackberries, raspberries, strawberries, oranges, lemons, apples, pears, bananas, grapes, cherries, kiwi fruit, watermelon, limes, pomegranate, mango

Dairy and Dairy Alternatives

Dairy (organic when possible)

Goat's cheese, sheep's cheese, plain unsweetened or naturally sweetened Greek Yogurt, Kefir

Dairy Alternatives

Rice milk, almond milk, hemp milk, coconut milk, organic or fermented soymilk, organic or fermented soy or coconut yogurt, vegan cheese

Good Fats/Oils – unrefined, cold-pressed oils

Organic butter or ghee (clarified butter), coconut oil, high oleic sunflower oil, sesame seed oil, extra-virgin olive oil, avocado oil, grape seed oil, flax seed oil, hemp seed oil

Vinegars/Sauces/Dressings

Unpasteurized apple cider vinegar, organic balsamic vinegar, rice vinegar, red wine vinegar, wheat-free soy sauce (Tamari or Braggs), and salad dressings without MSG or added sugar.

Flours

Brown rice flour, quinoa flour, buckwheat flour, 100% whole-wheat flour, millet flour, oat flour, coconut flour, chickpea flour

Sweeteners

Raw or manuka honey, pure maple syrup, stevia (liquid or powder), sucanat, molasses, cane juice, coconut sugar, brown rice syrup

Spices/Herbs/Seaweeds

Basil, bay leaves, rosemary, turmeric, chili pepper, coriander, fenugreek, chives, black pepper, cardamom, cayenne, nutmeg, oregano, parsley (fresh), cinnamon, cloves, black pepper, cumin, sea salt, thyme, dill (fresh), fennel seeds, garlic (fresh and/or powder), ginger (fresh and/or powder), mustard seeds

<u>Seaweeds</u>

Kelp, kombu, arame, wakame, nori

Other/Superfoods/Supplements

Baking powder, baking soda, carob powder, raw cocoa powder, xanthan gum, applesauce (unsweetened), cacao nibs or powder, sauerkraut (fermented), sea salt, pure vanilla extract, vegetable or chicken stock, nutritional yeast, mustard, goji berries, spirulina powder, matcha green tea powder, wheatgrass, aloe vera juice or gel, probiotics, fish oil, magnesium powder, dried unsweetened coconut, grape skin powder.

<u>Dried Fruit</u>

Dates, prunes, figs, dried cranberries, currants, unsulphured raisins - **All dried fruit should be unsweetened, without sulfites**

Beverages and Herbal Teas (loose leaf tea)

Ginger tea, rooibos tea, chamomile tea, dandelion tea, peppermint tea, lavender tea, licorice tea, and coconut water

GUNK-FILLED FOODS TO AVOID

- **Refined sugar, artificial sweeteners, and foods containing:** sucrose, maltose, lactose, glucose, mannitol, galactose, sorbitol, corn syrup, white sugar, aspartame, acesulfame-K
- **Fruit:** Candied, canned, bottled or frozen juices (very high in sugar and very acidic).
- **Dairy and Oil:** Cow's milk, butter, flavored or sweetened yogurt, cream, sour cream, ice cream (made with cow's milk), cheese made from cow's milk (especially processed cheese), blue cheese, cottage and cream cheese, margarine, hydrogenated vegetable oils, shortening, cooking sprays, and creamy dips.
- **Grains:** All products made with white flour. Bread, pasta, rice, cereals, muffins, cookies, cakes.
  - » Those with gluten-sensitivities, Celiac disease, those who experience digestive upset after consuming gluten-containing foods, or those who simply wish to go gluten-free should avoid: wheat, rye, barley, spelt, oats (other than gluten-free oats).
- **Processed and packaged snack foods** made with refined sugar, hydrogenated oil, white flour, artificial flavors, artificial sweeteners, monosodium glutamate, artificial colors and dyes.
- **Breaded and deep-fried foods,** unless homemade and breaded with whole grains and healthy oils.
- **Processed deli meat:** sausage, bacon, hot dogs, corned beef, pastrami, ham, turkey, bologna, and all other processed meats.
- **Condiments:** White vinegar, ketchup, pickled products (unless fermented), mayonnaise, bottled salad dressings (unless 100% natural), and barbeque sauce.
- **Any food containing:** monosodium glutamate (MSG, yeast extract, calcium glutamate), artificial color, dyes, artificial flavoring, hydrogenated oil, preservatives, saturated and trans fat, excess sodium, or refined sugar. *See page 2 for words to look for on product labels.*

- **Soy** (except for edamame or fermented soy) – *See page 76 for more on soy.*
- **Limit coffee and alcohol**
- **ALL FOODS TO WHICH YOU ARE SENSITIVE OR ALLERGIC.**

> Dairy is highly inflammatory and can be allergenic for many people. It is suggested to avoid dairy, especially cow's dairy, for at least a twenty-one day period to see whether or not dairy is something that negatively affects you. After that time, incorporating cow dairy back into your diet is optional. If you experience symptoms of gas, bloating, constipation, diarrhea, or digestive upset, adopting a dairy-free lifestyle long-term may be beneficial. *See page 57 for more on dairy.*
>
> After at least twenty-one days dairy-free, those who are not sensitive or allergic to it, may begin to reintroduce the following:
>
> - Organic milk
> - Organic butter
> - Ghee
> - Cheese (except for processed cheese)
> - Yogurt (plain, unsweetened)

21 Simple Gunk-Free Habits

GUNK-FREE HABIT #1
Set Goals and Go After Them

> *"Learn from the past, set vivid, detailed goals for the future, and live in the only moment of time over which you have any control: now"* – Denis Waitley

Part of what can make us feel gunky inside are our own negative thoughts that tell us that we can't do something or that attempting to do it is going to be too hard or too much work. This type of thinking is what holds us back from achieving happiness and fulfilling our goals.

"Every time I lose weight I gain it back", "Eating healthy is too much work", "I don't have enough time to prepare healthy food", "My partner won't eat what I make, so what's the point?"

These are called excuses. Excuses hold you back. Being held back means not being able to achieve success and ultimately fulfill your goals. Not being able to fulfill your goals can lead to feeling gunky inside. You get the idea!

Now, we don't always achieve the goals we set for ourselves, and that's okay. But as long as we try our best and have realistic plans in place to fulfill them, that's all that matters.

In order to de-gunk the goal setting process to make it simple and achievable, simply follow these guidelines.

GUNK-FREE GOAL SETTING

1. **WHAT** - Decide what it is that you want to achieve.
2. **WHEN** - Choose a realistic amount of time that it will take to achieve your goal.
3. **HOW, WHERE AND WHO** - Write down a step-by-step plan on how you are going to achieve your goal, including the people, places and things you are going to need.
4. **WHY** – Determine why you want to achieve your goal.
5. Keep a list and refer to it daily. Make any notes on your progress (or lack of) each day.
6. Do not let rejection or small mishaps deter you from powering through. Learn from any mistakes you make along the way, and make any necessary changes to your initial plan. Once you have achieved your goal (and you will), celebrate!

GUNK-FREE GOAL PLANNER

WHAT are your major goals?

1. _____
2. _____
3. _____

WHEN would you realistically like to achieve each goal by?

1. _____
2. _____
3. _____

> For a FREE, detailed, step-by-step goal planning and tracking journal, visit:
>
> shannonkadlovski.com

WHY do you want to achieve these goals?

1. _____
2. _____
3. _____

How do you feel about starting on this journey? (Nervous, excited, scared, etc.) Why?

_____

_____

HOW, WHERE AND WHO? What steps are you going to take to achieve your goals, and who and what are you going to need?

Goal #1	Goal #2	Goal #3
_____	_____	_____
_____	_____	_____
_____	_____	_____
_____	_____	_____

I am ready to commit to my health and work to achieve my goals.

_____   _____
Signature   Date

GUNK-FREE HABIT #2
Cut The Coffee and Cola and Sip on Some Tea

> **HABIT #2 HOW-TO:**
>
> **For coffee drinkers:** Completely eliminate coffee consumption for any consecutive twenty-one day period. Slowly reduce your intake of coffee to avoid withdrawal symptoms. If you normally drink three coffees per day, reduce to two for a few days, then to one, then to none. Or, reduce the size of your cup each day, having less and less as the days go on. Replace your coffee intake with green or herbal teas, maca, yerba mate, or other coffee alternatives. Giving yourself a twenty-one day (at least) break from coffee will help to eliminate dependency and turn future coffee drinking into an enjoyable practice rather than an addictive behavior.
>
> **For non-coffee drinkers:** Increase your intake of green or herbal teas, and try including maca into your diet.
>
> **For all:** Completely eliminate soda from your diet.

WHAT? ARE YOU CRAZY? YOU MEAN I HAVE TO START MY DAY WITHOUT COFFEE?

Wouldn't it be nice to be able to function without coffee? Overtime, your body becomes addicted to caffeine, making it harder and harder for you to get through the day without it. You experience fatigue, headaches, and mood swings when you don't get your coffee fix, and the only way to make yourself feel better is to reach for your favourite brew.

It is possible, however, to retrain your body so that you are no longer dependent on coffee, and better yet, retrain your body to not only not need it, but to feel fabulous without it.

The caffeine found in both coffee and soda can severely disrupt the nervous system and lead to anxiety, mood swings, and irritability. In addition, both coffee and soda displace many vitamins and minerals in the body, lead to dehydration, cause digestive issues, lead to insomnia, and the list goes on.

Most coffee beans are processed by drying them in the sun, which causes them to spoil as they sit out. Another method presses them, allowing them to go bad in order to remove the outer layer of the bean. The processing of coffee beans is known to produce high levels of mycotoxins (toxins that are produced from mold).

Now, this does not mean that you should never have a cup of coffee. Everything in moderation is key. However, it is important to understand the difference between enjoying a warm cup of coffee with friends, versus not being able to get through the day when your local morning coffee shop happens to be closed. It is the overconsumption and dependency that we want to avoid. If you are going to consume coffee on an occasional basis, it is essential to choose organic coffee.

I know what you're thinking...why can't I just drink decaf then, right?

The truth is, that decaffeinated coffee carries many of the same negative effects as regular coffee. For one thing, decaffeinated coffee still contains some traces of caffeine. By law, up to 2.5% of caffeine is allowed to remain in a product for it to be labeled "decaffeinated".

Decaffeinated coffee beans also contain the same amount of acidity as regular coffee beans. This over stimulates the digestive tract and causes imbalances within the intestinal system. It also prevents the body from absorbing various minerals such as iron, magnesium, and calcium as well as induces heartburn and acid reflux.

Many of the negative consequences associated with coffee consumption come from the actual coffee bean itself, not just the caffeine.

WHY IS SODA POP SO BAD?

Soda pop is extremely high in sugar, high in calories, and devoid of any nutrients. Most soft drinks contain high fructose corn syrup, caffeine, phosphoric acid, citric acid, and artificial flavors. All of these ingredients are harmful to our bodies in several ways.

High concentration of fructose sweeteners and phosphoric acid can cause calcium loss and weaken our bones. High fructose corn syrup can contribute to weight gain, dental cavities, and increased triglyceride levels. The amount of sugar found in these drinks simply adds extra empty calories to our diet.

Consuming too much phosphoric acid can affect the proper functioning of our kidneys. Many of the ingredients in soft drinks can increase the risk of gastrointestinal distress, resulting in uncomfortable stomach pains.

Drinking carbonated beverages, such as soda, adds air into your digestive system. This can lead to gas and bloating.

IS DIET POP A HEALTHY ALTERNATIVE?

Many people believe that choosing a diet beverage is a suitable alternative to regular soda. The reality is, that diet soda is equally as bad, if not worse for us, than regular soda. Diet soda contains the same ingredients as regular soda, but in addition, is filled with harmful artificial sweeteners, including aspartame. These artificial sweeteners have numerous negative effects on the body, including increased risk for heart disease, stroke and cancer. They are known to cause headaches, dizziness, migraines, nausea, anxiety, depression and difficulty breathing. Artificial sweeteners are known as an "excitotoxins", and can contribute to neurological disorders such as Parkinson's, MS, Alzheimer's, Lupus and Fibromyalgia. Artificial sweeteners have also been proven to over stimulate our appetite, causing us to eat more than we otherwise would have.

REPLACING COFFEE

Part of what we love so much about drinking coffee is the warm, comforting feeling it provides. Once you eliminate coffee from your diet, you may feel that you still want some kind of warm drink to soothe and comfort. The best options are yerba mate, maca, green tea or herbal tea. Even those who do not drink coffee can benefit from the amazing healing properties of these items.

Coffee-Like Blends

Many coffee-like blends are made from dandelion root, chicory, barley, and rye, and very closely resemble the taste of coffee without the negative effects associated with coffee consumption.

Suggested brands: Dandy blend, A Vogel, Teecino

Yerba Mate

- Yerba mate is made from the leaves of the holly tree.
- It is naturally caffeinated.
- It provides the boost of energy that coffee does, combined with the health benefits of tea.
- Rich in antioxidants, vitamins and minerals.
- Unlike coffee, yerba mate is not acid forming. Therefore, it is less likely to cause digestive upset and irritability.
- Can be consumed much like tea and coffee, with added milk alternative (rice milk, hemp milk, almond milk) and natural sweetener (honey, stevia, sucanat).

Maca

Maca is a cruciferous root known to provide energy, strength and endurance, and can be used as a coffee substitute. It can also be consumed by non-coffee drinkers for an extra boost of energy, and can be added to smoothies, used in baked goods, added to soups, dips and dressings.

Maca is not only a substitute for coffee, but is also considered a superfood (more superfoods on page 101), as it provides many health benefits. Maca is known to increase libido and fertility, as well as provide a source of energy. It provides the pick-me-up you seek without the negative side effects of coffee, such as jitters, energy crashes, and headaches. It helps to improve concentration and endurance. Maca is considered an adaptogen, which supports our adrenal glands and helps us cope with stress. Due to its balancing effect, maca can help balance our hormones, and in turn, help with symptoms of PMS, menopause and hot flashes.

Maca As A Coffee Substitute

Maca coffee blends do not actually contain any coffee, but are prepared in a way that gives off a coffee-like flavour. Some maca coffees are blended with other herbs, while others use only pure maca.

Pure maca powder can be added to hot water and consumed the same way as coffee (you can add some stevia or coconut sugar to sweeten, as well as your favourite dairy milk alternative – see page 61). Maca can also be added to cold beverages such as smoothies or cold lattes (with your favourite milk alternative).

Other Uses for Maca

- Add 1 tsp. to soup.
- Top your popcorn with it: combine 1 tsp. maca powder, 2 tbsp. coconut oil, and a pinch of sea salt.
- Add ½ tsp. to your tea.

If you are pregnant or have high blood pressure, consult your health care provider before using maca.

Green Tea

- Green tea contains potent antioxidants that help to protect the body against free-radical damage – thus acting as a cancer fighter.

21 SIMPLE GUNK-FREE HABITS   31

- It has been shown to help lower "bad" cholesterol (LDL) levels and aid with weight loss. This helps to protect against diabetes and heart disease.
- It helps to reduce inflammation associated with Crohn's disease and ulcerative colitis.
- Green tea helps to control blood sugar levels.
- Although caffeinated, it is milder than coffee and does not lead to the same jittery feeling that coffee can.
- Consume one to two cups of green tea daily.
- Always choose loose-leaf green tea.

Matcha Green Tea Powder

- Matcha is a premium green tea powder from Japan.
- It is often used as a warm beverage or added to recipes.
- Matcha has a rich, astringent, yet sweet taste.
- It is extremely rich in nutrients, antioxidants and chlorophyll, which help to prevent oxidative stress in the body, as well and cleanse and detoxify the kidneys, liver and digestive system.
- Matcha is completely sugar-free.
- It contains caffeine, but provides a steady source of energy, while also helping to relax the mind and body.

How Matcha Differs From Green Tea

- When consuming matcha, the whole leaf is ingested, not just the brewed water, as is the case for green tea. One serving of matcha is equivalent to ten servings of green tea in terms of nutrition and antioxidant content.

Using Matcha

- Mix 1 tsp. matcha with six ounces hot water and consume much the same way as any other tea.
- It can be added to smoothies, dessert recipes, yogurt, homemade ice cream, or sauces.

Herbal Teas

Herbal teas are a great substitute for caffeinated beverages. Not only are they free of caffeine, but they also have many incredible health benefits. They can be consumed as an alternative to coffee, or simply as part of a healthy, gunk-free diet.

Ginger tea

- Reduces inflammation in the joints.
- Assists in proper digestion.
- Improves blood flow and encourages normal blood circulation.
- Contains antioxidants that help strengthen the immune system.
- Improves mood and relieves stress.

Dandelion tea

- Purifies blood and cleanses system.
- Aids digestion.
- Helps to reduce high cholesterol.
- Improves the function of and maintains optimum liver, kidney, pancreas, spleen, and stomach.
- Helps with weight control.

Rooibos tea

- Contain high level of antioxidants that help fight off free radicals and keep our bodies healthy.
- Helps with insomnia, tension, headaches and irritability.
- Contains high levels of manganese, fluoride and calcium, which promote stronger bones and teeth.
- Aids digestion – helps with nausea, heartburn and constipation.

Peppermint tea

- Prevents build up of gas in the digestive tract.
- Soothes feeling of nausea and helps to prevent urge to vomit.

- Strengthens immune system.
- Helps break down gallstones.
- Helps reduce stress.
- Can aid headaches and aid in a restful sleep.

Chamomile tea

- Aids in restful sleep.
- Eases symptoms of IBS, promotes regular bowel movements and aids in overall proper digestion.
- Helps combat menstrual cramps.
- Strengthens the immune system.

Lavender tea

- Can be used as treatment for insomnia and restless sleep.
- Soothes migraines and headaches.
- Relieves indigestion.
- Can be effective for reducing anxiety and stress.
- Can help alleviate respiratory disorders.

Licorice tea

- Stress relief and anti-depressant.
- Helps to lower cholesterol.
- Anti-inflammatory properties, which help ease pain from arthritis.
- Can help prevent heart disease.
- Protects stomach tissue and reduces symptoms of stomach upset and ulcers.
- Has a diuretic effect - eases water retention and build up of toxins.

Choose loose-leaf tea over conventional tea bags. Loose-leaf tea contains whole, unbroken leaves, giving the tea a much richer and fresher flavour. It also helps to retain many of the nutrients and benefits that the tea provides, as it has not been heavily processed and broken down.

SUMMARY

<u>For coffee drinkers</u>

- Slowly reduce your intake of coffee until you no longer require coffee on a daily basis.
- Do not drink any coffee for a consecutive twenty-one day period in order to eliminate the dependency.
- When drinking coffee in moderation, opt for an organic brew.
- Replace coffee with yerba mate, maca, green or herbal teas, or other coffee alternatives.
- Completely eliminate soda from your diet.

<u>For non-coffee drinkers</u>

- Increase your intake of green or herbal teas and try to include maca in your diet.
- Completely eliminate soda from your diet.

GUNK-FREE HABIT #3
Lose the Booze

> **HABIT #3 HOW-TO:** Limit alcohol intake on a regular basis. In addition, choose any consecutive twenty-one day period to avoid alcohol altogether. This will give your body and your liver a much-needed break.

Consuming alcohol makes getting the gunk out of your body very difficult. Our bodies see alcohol as a toxin, so continuing to consume it while trying to de-gunk your body is extremely counter intuitive.

If you choose to consume alcohol, do so in moderation. If you normally consume alcohol three to four times per week, try to reduce that number to one or two. If you normally consume beer, for example, trying opting for a glass of red wine or clear liquor once in a while instead (or completely replace your beer consumption with it). Or, better yet, give up the booze on a regular basis and choose to drink only at parties, social gatherings or other events. Leave it for those special occasions.

WHY WE'RE GIVING UP THE BOOZE

Your Liver Needs A Break

The liver takes a serious beating when it comes to alcohol consumption. Although the liver contains specific enzymes that break down alcohol into other chemicals before entering the body, drinking too much alcohol puts a burden on the liver. We need our livers to help remove toxins from the body, and it can only do so when it is not overwhelmed with alcohol and other toxins. Alcohol simply interferes with the detoxification process and the livers ability to do its job.

Your Digestive System Will Thank You

Alcohol delays stomach emptying time, causing gas, pain, bloating, and fat storage. Therefore, drinking alcohol with a meal is incredibly hard on your digestive system. The body recognizes alcohol as a toxin and therefore focuses on breaking it down first, while neglecting to break down carbohydrates and protein from the food you are eating. These items get stored as fat instead of being used for energy, as the body cannot work to break them down properly in the presence of alcohol.

You Deserve Some Good Quality Sleep

Alcohol affects the quality of your sleep. Depending on how much alcohol you have consumed, you may find that falling asleep is very easy. However, as the night goes on, you may notice that you begin to toss and turn – resulting in a very restless sleep. This is because alcohol affects the second half of our sleep cycle, causing restlessness and wakefulness. The lack of good quality sleep while intoxicated can lead to feeling tired, groggy and "off" the following day. The closer to bedtime alcohol is consumed, the worse the second half of our sleep is.

Try kombucha in place of alcohol. This fermented tea has a fizzy texture and tastes like a sparkling apple cider or champagne. It helps promote proper digestion, aids with weight loss, boosts energy, and helps to cleanse the liver.

SUMMARY

- Limit alcohol on a regular basis.
- Choose any twenty-one day period to go completely booze-free.
- When consuming alcohol, do so in moderation.
- Opt for clear alcohol or red wine instead of beer.
- Avoid drinking a few hours before going to sleep, as this can make for a very restless, poor-quality sleep.
- Avoid drinking alcohol with your meal. It prevents the proper breakdown of your food and can lead to digestive upset.

GUNK-FREE HABIT #4
Replace Refined Sugar

> **HABIT #4 HOW-TO**: Replace all refined sugar (including products made with it) with healthier, natural alternatives such as pure maple syrup, raw honey, sucanat, stevia, molasses, and dates.

Have a sweet tooth? No need to worry. Just because you're cutting out white, refined sugar from your diet doesn't mean you won't be able to indulge in delicious, sweet snacks. So, you can still have your cake and eat it too!

WHAT IS REFINED SUGAR AND WHY IS IT SO BAD?

Refined sugar is one of the most common ingredients found in processed and packaged foods. It can be found in a wide variety of foods including breakfast cereals, sweets (cookies, chocolate bars, snack packs, ice cream, cake, and candy), breads, pastries, soups, pasta sauces, juices, soft drinks, dressings, and other condiments. Many people also add it to coffee, tea, or other drinks, and commonly include it in cooking or baking.

Refined sugar is the "white" stuff. White sugar has been put through a refining process, which strips it of all vitamins and minerals. It is a completely nutrient void substance that provides empty calories and contributes to weight gain, diabetes, mood swings, anxiety, and a host of other symptoms. Consuming white sugar leads to food cravings, which send you back to the cupboard for more sugary foods. In order to eliminate these cravings and prevent overeating, we must eliminate all white sugar (including products containing it), from the diet.

WHAT ABOUT BROWN SUGAR?

Brown sugar is still sugar, even though it's brown. It comes with all of the negative effects that white sugar does, as it is just as heavily processed and nutrient void. The only benefit of brown sugar over white sugar is that it has a little bit of its molasses content in tact – giving it its brown color. Brown sugar, along with the "white stuff", has got to go.

THE EFFECTS OF REFINED SUGAR ON OUR HEALTH

Consuming refined sugar has a major impact on our blood sugar levels and overall health. It is important to understand what happens inside our bodies when we consume refined sugar.

- When we ingest refined sugar, our blood glucose levels rise.
- This causes the pancreas to release insulin (which is responsible for lowering blood sugar to a safe level).
- The sugar is then diverted to the liver and tissues to be used as energy or stored as fat.
- If, however, there is an over-release of insulin (from consuming too much sugar, too frequently), blood sugar levels can fall too low.
- When this happens, we experience headaches, irritability, fatigue, nausea, and are unable to focus. We also begin to crave more sugar and refined carbohydrates in order to bring our blood sugar levels back up to normal, and often dive head first into the cookie jar or tub of ice cream.
- This cycle continues to repeat itself over and over again, resulting in cravings and overconsumption of refined carbohydrates.
- Eventually, if this goes on for long enough, the sugar consumed continues to get stored as fat, which leads to obesity and even diabetes (where the pancreas can no longer function and do its job).
- Even though refined sugar gives us energy temporarily, it eventually results in an energy crash and the need for more sugar. A vicious cycle.

Sugar consumption can also impact our physical appearance. The bacteria in our mouths use sugar in our diet to form substances that cause tooth decay. Refined sugar also robs the body of calcium and other minerals, causing our bones to weaken. This may lead to conditions such as osteoporosis or arthritis.

ARTIFICIAL SWEETENERS

Artificial sweeteners are synthetic sugar substitutes. They are many times sweeter than regular sugar and do not contain any calories. Some common artificial sweeteners include acesulfame potassium, aspartame (NutraSweet, Equal), saccharin (Sweet'N Low), cyclamate (SugarTwin), and sucralose (Splenda).

Although artificial sweeteners do not cause spikes in insulin or contain any calories, they must be avoided. They are filled with chemicals that contribute to headaches, dizziness, nausea, anxiety, depression, and have even been linked to heart disease and cancer. In addition, artificial sweeteners have actually been known to lead to more sugar and carbohydrate cravings. So, even though we are saving ourselves a few calories now, we end up eating more throughout the day.

IDENTIFYING SUGAR ON FOOD LABELS

The following is a list of possible code words for sugar, which may appear on a product label. These are the ones we want to AVOID. In addition, anything ending in "ose" is typically sugar.

- Barley malt syrup
- Corn sweetener
- Corn syrup, or corn syrup solids
- Dextrin
- Dextrose
- Fructose
- Fruit juice concentrate
- Glucose
- High-fructose corn syrup
- Invert sugar
- Maltodextrin
- Malt syrup
- Saccharose
- Sucrose
- Treacle
- Turbinado sugar

REPLACING REFINED SUGAR – HEALTHIER ALTERNATIVES

Eating healthy doesn't mean having to give up sweets - it simply means choosing the right types of natural sweeteners. Just because you are eliminating refined sugar from your daily diet, does not mean that all sweets need to be avoided. There are plenty of natural alternatives that are much healthier.

Dates

- Good source of fiber, as well as many essential vitamins and minerals.
- Help to relieve constipation and promote proper bowel function.
- Good source of potassium.
- Quick source of energy, but do not make us feel sluggish and tired the same way refined sugar can.
- Promote the growth of friendly, beneficial bacteria in the intestines.
- Increase sexual stamina.

* Add to smoothies, baked goods, trail mixes or consume on their own as part of a healthy snack.

Raw Honey

- Raw honey has not been processed or pasteurized in any way.
- Contains bee pollen and propolis (which the bees use to protect their hives and prevent bacteria and viruses from invading).
- Soothing for our throats and helps to protect our immune systems.

* Add to tea, baked goods, smoothies, oatmeal, or salad dressings.

To replace 1 cup white sugar with honey – Use ¾ cup honey. When baking with honey, reduce other liquid ingredients in the recipe by three tablespoons.

Pure Maple Syrup

- Does not contain coloring agents, artificial flavorings or other additives and is 100% natural.
- It is rich in magnesium, riboflavin, zinc, magnesium and calcium.
- It is important to note that pure maple syrup is very different than other liquid "syrups". These syrups are made from liquid sugar, artificial flavours, caramel color, sulfites and other unhealthy ingredients that must be avoided.
- Make sure the bottle says 100% pure maple syrup with no other ingredients listed.

* Use pure maple syrup on whole grain pancakes, baked goods, marinades, and salad dressings.

To replace one cup white sugar with pure maple syrup – Use ¾ cup pure maple syrup. When baking with maple syrup, reduce other liquid ingredients in the recipe by three tablespoons.

Sucanat

- Sucanat is unrefined, evaporated cane sugar.
- Does cause spikes in insulin levels, but is much richer in vitamins and minerals than refined white sugar.

* It can be used the same way white sugar is used.

To replace one cup white sugar with sucanat – Use one cup sucanat (a 1:1 ratio).

Molasses

- Produced when cane sugar is refined into white sugar. It is what is left over after the refining process.
- Great source of iron, potassium, magnesium, calcium and selenium.

To replace one cup white sugar with molasses – Use 1 1/3 cups molasses. When baking with molasses, reduce other liquid ingredients in the recipe by five tablespoons.

Stevia

- Stevia comes from the stevia plant and is natural and calorie-free.
- It contains vitamins and minerals and is also said to have anti-microbial properties.
- Stevia does not affect blood sugar levels and is therefore safe for diabetics.
- Stevia can be purchased in leaf, powder or liquid form.
- Stevia is almost 300 times sweeter than table sugar, so you do not need to use as much.

* Can be used to sweeten beverages, in baking, or wherever else sugar is used.

To replace one cup white sugar with stevia – Use one to two teaspoons stevia.

GUNK-FREE SWEET TREATS

Whoever said that eating healthy meant having to give up sweets was sadly mistaken. Not only do we not have to give up sweets, but many of the gunk-free snack and dessert recipes that you are about to indulge in are made with wholesome, nourishing, mood boosting, and energy intensifying ingredients. So, eat that, naysayers!

As mentioned previously, the types of sweeteners that we are using cause less severe spikes in our blood sugar levels, contain many vitamins and minerals, and do not contribute to the same negative effects that refined sugar does. That being said, it is still important to not over-indulge in sweet snacks. The beautiful thing about gunk-free snacks is that they leave us feeling satisfied, rather than craving more and more sweets. So, having just one is often enough.

See page 204 for delicious, gunk-free sweet treat recipes.

STORE BOUGHT SNACKS

The truth is, that sometimes with busy schedules and barely enough time to make the bed in the morning, making your own snacks is simply not an option. We get busy and even lazy sometimes, and that's okay. The good news is that there are plenty of healthy snacks on the market made with ingredients that not only taste delicious, but are also really good for us.

What Does A Healthy Store-Bought Snack Look Like?

When purchasing store bought snacks, avoid being drawn in by fancy marketing slogans, but instead look directly at the list of ingredients. If the ingredient label includes refined sugar, hydrogenated oils, refined flour, artificial flavors and coloring, monosodium glutamate (MSG), or high fructose corn syrup, simply put it down and move on to the next.

Look for snacks made with whole grains, natural sweeteners, nuts, seeds, healthy oils, and spices.

For a list of suggested store-bought snack brands see page 215.

SUMMARY

- Eliminate white "refined" sugar from your diet.
- Avoid brown sugar, as it is simply white sugar with molasses added back.
- Avoid artificial sweeteners at all costs.
- Make sure to read food labels to identify key words that indicate refined sugar. Words ending in "ose" typically mean sugar.
- Replace refined sugar in your diet with natural alternatives such as dates, pure maple syrup, raw honey, molasses, stevia, and sucanat.
- Make your own sweet snacks at home or purchase store-bought gunk-free snacks.

GUNK-FREE HABIT #5
Get More Whole Grains

> **HABIT #5 HOW-TO:** Replace refined "white" carbohydrates in your diet with whole grains and other fiber-rich complex carbohydrates. Consume between 25-40 grams of fiber each day.

Often, we hear about fad diets that promote eliminating carbohydrates from the diet completely. And while eliminating refined "white" carbohydrates from the diet is highly beneficial, eliminating all carbohydrates, including whole grains, does more harm than good. Complex carbohydrates, including whole grains, legumes, and starchy vegetables provide the body with fuel and energy. They are needed for proper organ function and are an important part of a healthy diet.

WHAT ARE REFINED "BAD" CARBOHYDRATES?

Refined carbohydrates are foods that have been processed by machinery that strip the bran and germ (which provide a good source of fiber and other essential nutrients) from the whole grain. During the refining process, the bran and germ are removed, the grain is polished using glucose (sugar), and the end result is a nutrient void, fiber-deficient grain. This process helps to prolong shelf life and gives the food a finer texture, but all at the cost of our health. This process removes important nutrients, such as B vitamins, fiber, and iron, and causes these items to convert to sugar much quicker, causing sudden spikes in our blood sugar levels. They are filled with empty calories.

Refined carbohydrates are not good for us because they have what is called a high glycemic index. This means that these foods cause a sudden and sharp increase in blood sugar levels. This leads to cravings, energy crashes, and can even lead to obesity and diabetes over time.

Carbohydrates to Avoid

When choosing products, avoid those that are labeled as "made with" or "containing" whole grains. This indicates that the product is not a true whole grain product. **A true whole grain product will have the whole grain listed as the first or only ingredient.**

Avoid:
- White, refined or all purpose flour found in breads, bagel, pastries, cakes, cookies
- White rice
- White pasta
- White bread
- Couscous

WHAT ARE WHOLE GRAINS AND WHY ARE THEY GOOD FOR US?

Whole grains (or foods made from them) contain all of the essential parts and naturally occurring nutrients of the entire grain seed.

Some common whole grains include: Whole wheat, brown rice, whole corn, whole oats, whole rye, whole barley, quinoa, buckwheat, whole sorghum, and whole millet.

Benefits of Whole Grains

Cardiovascular health: Eating whole grains helps to lower total cholesterol and "bad" cholesterol, lower triglycerides, and helps to keep blood sugar levels stable. This can help to prevent and protect against cardiovascular disease.

Type II Diabetes and Weight Management: Whole grains have a relatively high fiber content. This helps to keep blood sugar levels balanced by slowing down the absorption of sugar into our bloodstream and therefore preventing significant spikes in insulin. The high fiber content also helps to keep you feeling fuller for longer, thus preventing overeating.

Digestive health: The fiber in whole grains helps to prevent constipation, and enables things to move properly inside your digestive system.

Whole Grains to Include in Your Diet

When choosing products such as rice, pasta, rice cakes, flours, crackers, breads and cereals, look for these words on the label:

- Steel cut oats or rolled oats
- 100% whole grain cereals (be careful of those that say "contains whole grains" – these items generally do not contain 100% whole grains)

- Whole wheat berries
- Whole wheat bulgur
- Kamut
- Spelt
- Brown rice
- Whole rye
- Hulled barley
- Triticale
- Millet
- Teff
- Buckwheat
- Quinoa
- Amaranth

Oats

Oats are a great source of fiber, which helps to promote healthy digestion. They are absorbed slowly in the body, thus providing us with sustained energy and satiety. Oats also work to balance blood sugar levels, and are therefore beneficial for preventing or managing diabetes. They are a great source of soluble fiber, which has been shown to help lower cholesterol. They are incredibly high in calcium, potassium, magnesium, and B vitamins, which are all vital to a healthy nervous system.

Using Oats

- **Steel cut oats** are the least processed type of oat. They must be cooked in order to be enjoyed. Cook for approximately ten minutes.
- **Rolled oats** require less cooking time. They can be consumed right out of the bag (in a raw desert recipe or added to smoothies),

or cooked in water for approximately three to five minutes, and enjoyed as a hot cereal.

- **Oat bran** is made from the outer shell of the oat kernel. It is available as a finely ground meal which is delicious when cooked as a hot cereal. Oat bran can also be used in baking. When consuming oat bran as a hot cereal, top with some pure maple syrup and fresh berries for a bit of sweetness.
- **Avoid quick oats**, as they are the most heavily processed. They have been chopped, flattened, and pre-cooked, and are typically made with added salt and sugar. It is recommended to avoid quick oats.

* *Rolled oats are a great, high fiber substitution for breadcrumbs. When making a homemade breaded chicken, use rolled oats in place of breadcrumbs.*

> **Gunk-Free Tip:** Make a large batch of steel cut or rolled oats and store in the fridge for up to four days. For breakfast, simply scoop out a portion and reheat on the stovetop for three to five minutes. This makes for a healthy, high-fiber breakfast in minutes.

Quinoa

Don't be fooled by its funny and somewhat unpronounceable name – quinoa (pronounced keen-wa) is one of the most delicious and nutritious foods around.

Quinoa is a whole grain and is incredibly high in protein. In fact, it is a complete protein, as it contains all of the essential amino acids our bodies need. It is a great source of fiber, which helps to promote proper elimination and digestive function. Quinoa is also very high in magnesium, which helps to relax our nervous system. Quinoa helps to keep us feeling full for longer and keeps our blood sugar balanced. It is also gluten-free.

Using Quinoa

Rinse quinoa thoroughly. Bring two cups of water to a boil and add one cup of quinoa. Cover and cook on medium for twelve minutes (until all of the water is absorbed). Remove from heat and let stand for fifteen minutes.

Can be eaten hot or cold – for breakfast, lunch or dinner. Can be consumed the same way as rice or couscous.

Delicious quinoa recipes on pages 193 and 195.

Store cooked quinoa in the refrigerator for up to four days. Uncooked quinoa should be stored in an airtight container.

OTHER COMPLEX CARBOHYDRATES TO INCLUDE IN YOUR DIET

Whole grains are part of the family of complex carbohydrates, and while consuming whole grains each day is essential, it is also important to consume other types of complex carbohydrates as well.

Starchy Vegetables

Starchy vegetables are great sources of vitamins, minerals and fiber. Try some of the following:

- Parsnip
- Pumpkin
- Sweet potato
- Acorn squash
- Butternut squash
- Green Peas
- Corn (non-GMO, organic)

Legumes

Legumes include beans, peas and lentils. They are a great source of protein, which helps to reduce sugar cravings and nourish our muscles. They are high in fiber, as well as many vitamins and minerals. They are extremely beneficial for lowering levels of "bad" cholesterol and significantly help to reduce total cholesterol. They are filling and help to prevent overeating.

They provide a slow burning source of energy, which helps to stabilize blood sugar and helps to keep us feeling great throughout the day.

Legumes to Include In Your Diet
- Black, lima, kidney and pinto beans
- Lentils
- Black-eyed peas and split peas
- Garbanzo beans (chickpeas)
- Mung beans
- Edamame (soybeans)

When purchasing beans and legumes, the best option is to purchase them raw and cook them yourself. If you do not have the time to cook your own, purchase canned varieties with no added sodium. Look for brands that come in BPA-free cans and contain kombu in place of salt.

Kombu is a sea vegetable, rich in minerals, vitamins and natural glutamic salts, making it a great flavoring agent. It is often used in products as well as in cooking in place of salt.

Beans, lentils and peas can be served in a variety of different ways. For example, chickpeas may be added to salads, used to make a spread (hummus recipe on page 182), or as part of a soup. Different types of legumes can also be used to make chili dishes or stews. Try adding your favorite legumes to a salad, or serve with any meat or fish dish.

Using Legumes

Canned - Watch out for canned varieties with added salt. Look for organic, low sodium beans, in BPA free cans.

Dried - Cook one cup of dry beans in four cups of water. Bring them to a boil and reduce to a simmer for one to two hours, partially covered. Can store cooked beans in the fridge for up to four days in a covered container.

Gunk-Free Tip: To shorten cooking time and make them easier to digest, beans should be pre-soaked. Place them in a saucepan and add two to three cups of water per cup of beans. Soak for four to eight hours, rinse, and place into a saucepan with fresh water, to be cooked. Adding some kombu to the pot while cooking will also help to reduce cooking time and add some extra flavour.

FIBER MAKES US FEEL POOP-TASTIC!

Happy bowels equal happy life. It is important to consume adequate fiber in order to promote proper bowel function, cleanse the digestive system, and balance blood sugar levels.

Fiber helps to keep our bowels happy, and when our bowels are happy, the rest of our body is happy. Getting adequate fiber in our diet is incredibly important, but how much fiber do we really need? **It is recommended to consume between 25-40 grams of fiber each day.** Simply adding good quality, fiber-rich foods to each meal will enable you to meet your daily fiber needs.

Fiber has so many great health benefits - It helps to keep us feeling full for longer and is therefore great for weight loss. It also helps to keep blood sugar balanced by slowing down the absorption of sugar into our bloodstream, and prevents crashes in energy levels. Fiber also helps to lower cholesterol, improve bowel function and reduce the risk of colon cancer.

Our digestive system is one of our major pathways for elimination and detoxification. In order to help promote cleaning of the digestive system, we need to make sure we are consuming enough fiber to keep things moving.

When introducing more fiber into your diet, always make sure to start slowly. Start with 10-15 grams per day and work your way up to between 25-40 grams over the span of one week. Doing so enables your body to adapt to the increased fiber intake and prevents symptoms such as gas, bloating and digestive upset.

Everybody poops. And in fact, a healthy person goes about three times per day. The general rule of thumb is that we should be going number two after each meal. Now, this is ideal, however, it is not always the case. If you are going more than three times per day, less than once every other day, or if your stools are extremely hard or extremely loose on a regular basis, this may be a sign of food intolerance or inflammation in the digestive system. Keep a close eye on your bowel habits and consult your medical practitioner if you notice any of these patterns.

So, how do we get more fiber in our diet? By consuming more plant foods!

Simple Tips for Getting More Fiber

Flaxseeds and chia seeds: Add 1-2 tbsp. of ground flax seeds or chia seeds to any meal or drink.

Note: Flax seeds must be ground in order to be properly digested. Do not eat them whole, as they will just go through your system completely intact and come out the other end. Purchase whole flaxseeds, and (using a coffee grinder or nut/seed grinder) grind the seeds and store in the fridge. Or, purchase pre-ground flaxseeds. **For more information on flaxseeds see page 103.**

Fruits and vegetables: Consume a variety of fresh fruits and vegetables including, Brussels sprouts, broccoli, carrots, apples, citrus fruit, peaches, plums, pears and celery. Consume vegetables at each meal.

Legumes: Consume a variety of legumes, which provide a great source of protein and fiber. These include, kidney beans, lima beans, chickpeas, lentils, and black-eyed peas.

Oats: Consume steel cut oats, rolled oats, and oat bran, which are a great source of fiber and will help to balance blood sugar.

100% Whole Grains: Consume a variety of whole grains, such as buckwheat, rye, brown rice, quinoa, and amaranth.

Raw Nuts and Seeds: Consume raw, unsalted, nuts and seeds. These include almonds, hazelnuts, pecans, cashews, pine nuts, Brazil nuts, sesame seeds, pumpkin seeds, flax seeds, chia seeds and hemp seeds.

> **Gunk-Free Tip:**
> If you suffer from nut allergies
> - Use seeds such as pumpkin seeds, sunflower seeds, sesame seeds, hemp seeds, flax seeds and chia seeds.
> - Use seed butters such as sunflower seed or sesame seed butter.
> - Those with allergies to peanuts, but not tree nuts, can try almond butter and cashew butter.

GLUTEN-FREE - IS THIS FOR ME?

Gluten is the protein found in wheat, rye, barley, spelt, kamut, semolina, triticale, faro and durum.

When we consume foods containing gluten, an immune reaction may occur, which gradually damages the villi (small hairs) in the small intestine. When this happens, the body is unable to absorb vitamins, minerals and other nutrients, and causes symptoms such as gas, bloating, diarrhea, lethargy, brain fog, abdominal pain, fatigue, and skin rashes. As the villi become damaged, and inflammation occurs, this is referred to as celiac disease.

Whether you have been diagnosed with celiac disease, or are simply gluten-sensitive (react to gluten containing foods, but do not suffer from the immune reaction or inflammation associated with celiac disease) it is best to adopt a gluten-free diet. In fact, anyone can benefit from eating this way, especially those who experience any of the symptoms listed above after consuming gluten-containing foods.

Adopting a gluten-free diet can help promote weight loss, improve digestion, and increase energy.

The Gluten-Free Trial

Whether you suffer from gluten sensitivity or not, or are simply unaware whether or not gluten is contributing to symptoms you may be experiencing, it is a good idea to adopt a completely gluten-free diet for at least a twenty-one day period. This helps to give your digestive system a break, as well as enables you to identify whether or not you have been sensitive to gluten and simply haven't realized it yet.

After only a few short days on a gluten-free diet, you may begin to feel great and symptom free. If this is the case, it is best to remain on a gluten-free diet long term, since overtime, symptoms can worsen and lead to further damage in the small intestine. If a complete gluten-free lifestyle is not for you, perhaps choose a few days per week or a few meals per week to go completely gluten-free. Even small steps and small changes can make an incredible difference in the quality of your health.

> **Gunk-Free Tip:**
> Grain-free, gluten-free options
> - Use broad leafy greens such as romaine lettuce, kale and Swiss chard to replace flour wraps. The broad leafy greens are perfect for filling with protein and veggies.
> - Try spaghetti squash in place of pasta – Cut squash in half and cook in the oven at 350°F in a glass baking dish, with some water, for about forty minutes. Once soft, use your fork to scoop out the spaghetti-like flesh.

Gluten-Free Grains to Consume

- Foods made with the flours of organic corn, brown rice, buckwheat, sorghum, coconut, arrowroot, garbanzo beans (chickpeas), quinoa, tapioca, teff, potato, and gluten-free oats.
- Use gluten-free pastas such as brown rice pasta, buckwheat pasta, organic corn pasta, or quinoa pasta.

Buckwheat – This fruit seed is not related to wheat despite its name. The roasted groats or kasha can be cooked the same as rice (one part buckwheat to two parts liquid). Buckwheat has a robust, earthy flavour and can be used as a stuffing in chicken, added to soups, or eaten as a side dish. Store in an airtight container in a cool, dry place for up to one year. Buckwheat is high in magnesium, manganese, and protein.

Brown rice and basmati rice make great stir-fries and side dishes. They contain B vitamins, selenium, and fiber.

Bean flours (chickpea flour, pinto bean flour) – These flours combine well with other gluten-free flours and work well in baking recipes, breads and even to thicken sauces. Store in a tightly sealed container in the fridge up to six months.

Arrowroot flour can be used to thicken sauces, soups, gravies and pudding. Store in a cool, dark location in a tightly sealed container.

Coconut flour has high protein content and is perfect for denser baked goods or thickening soups and stews.

Amaranth is high in magnesium, manganese, and fiber. Whole grain amaranth can be boiled in water and used as a cereal substitute or side dish.

Potato starch can be used in place of wheat flour to thicken gravies, sauces, and soups. It can be mixed with gluten-free flours in baked goods to provide lightness and stretch.

Flax seeds can be ground and sprinkled on salads, hot cereal or yogurt for additional fiber. It can also be mixed with water to make an egg substitute for baking. *More on flax on page 103.*

Sorghum flour is a great source of antioxidants and works well as a gluten-free flour substitute in baking and pizza crusts. If working with whole grain sorghum, soak overnight before using. Add one-part sorghum grains to two parts water and bring to a boil. After it boils, reduce to a simmer and cook for about fifty minutes.

Chia seeds are a great source of fiber, antioxidants, and omega-3 fatty acids. They can be sprinkled on toast, salads, hot cereal, and even added to smoothies. *More on chia on page 101.*

Gluten Containing Foods to Avoid

- All purpose flour
- Wheat flour
- Breads, bagels, croissants, buns (unless they say gluten-free)
- Beer
- Marinades, sauces, soy and teriyaki sauces (unless they say gluten-free)
- Luncheon and processed meats
- Malt or malt flavoring (usually made from barley)
- Prepared mustards
- Canned soup
- Coffee substitutes (some are made with barley)
- Items labeled wheat-free (wheat free does not mean gluten free; many wheat-free cookies and breads contain barley or rye flour, which contains gluten and other gluten-containing ingredients).

Do Oats Contain Gluten?

Although oats do not contain gluten, they do contain a similar protein called avenin. Some people are sensitive to this protein as well, and therefore, those who are sensitive commonly avoid oats altogether. Only a small percentage of individuals are affected with avenin sensitivity, however, those who are gluten-sensitive typically avoid oats due to their high gluten contamination rate. In some cases, wheat and other gluten-grains accidentally get into the oats, which can affect those who are gluten-intolerant or gluten-sensitive. When consuming oats, it is best to select ones that indicate that they are completely gluten-free.

> **Gunk-Free Tip:** Just because it says gluten-free does not mean it's healthy. Many gluten-free products contain refined sugar and other artificial ingredients. Always make sure to read the ingredients list before purchasing any packaged foods.

SUMMARY

- Avoid all refined grains including white rice, white pasta, couscous, white bread and baked goods.
- Consume more whole grains including: Brown rice, whole corn, whole oats, whole rye, whole barley, quinoa, buckwheat, whole sorghum, and whole millet.
- Consume starchy vegetables including: Pumpkin, corn (non GMO), squash, and sweet potato.
- Consume legumes including: Lentils, peas, chickpeas, kidney beans, edamame, and navy beans.
- Consume between 25-40 grams of fiber per day. Fiber-rich foods include: flax seeds, chia seeds, fresh fruits and vegetables, oats, whole grains, raw nuts and seeds, and legumes.
- If you are sensitive to gluten, avoid wheat, rye, spelt, barley and oats.
- Try adopting a gluten-free diet for at least twenty-one days in order to give your digestive system a break.
- Consider adopting a completely gluten-free lifestyle long term, or simply choose a few days per week or a few meals per week to go completely gluten-free.

GUNK-FREE HABIT #6
No More Moo

Many people are sensitive to dairy, and an overwhelming part of the population suffers from lactose intolerance and/or dairy allergies. Many people experience symptoms associated with dairy consumption, such as digestive upset, inflammation, excess mucus, and congestion, yet do not relate the two, and continue to consume it.

> **HABIT #6 HOW-TO:** Making the choice to go completely dairy-free for at least twenty-one days will help to de-gunk your body and improve digestive function. You may notice that you have more energy, your skin begins to clear up, your nose becomes clear, and you experience less gas, bloating and headaches. If this happens, that is a very good indicator that dairy has been contributing to increased inflammation and mucous production in your body. After the twenty-one days, re-introduce dairy into your diet and see how you feel. If congestion and symptoms of irritable bowel return, you may want to consider adopting a dairy-free lifestyle long-term.

Between the ages of two to five, we naturally stop producing substantial amounts of lactase - the enzyme needed to metabolize lactose (the sugar found in milk). This means that our bodies are no longer equipped to properly digest milk, which can lead to symptoms such as gas, bloating, diarrhea, abdominal pain, sinus infections, excess mucous production, and acne. In addition to lactose, milk contains the protein casein, which often passes through the digestive tract undigested, also contributing to digestive distress.

Since everyone is different, and this book is about choosing your own wellness path, it is up to you to decide whether or not a dairy-free lifestyle is something that you would like to adopt. That being said, it is important to understand the facts about dairy, in order to make an informed decision.

DAIRY AND YOUR HEALTH

Research done on the negative effects of dairy on our health indicate that consuming cow dairy can lead to digestive problems, weakening of the bones, heart disease and even cancer. According to Dr. T. Colin Campbell, professor emeritus of nutritional biochemistry at Cornell University and author of The China Study, casein (the protein found in dairy) is one of the most significant cancer promoters. In addition, dairy products are high in cholesterol and saturated fat, which can contribute to heart disease.

HORMONES, ANTIBIOTICS AND YOU

Here's the deal - If your milk comes from a cow, there is a very good chance that it contains growth hormones and/or antibiotics. And while you will never meet that cow, and may not be concerned about what it has been fed or the conditions in which it lives, the truth is, that as soon as you drink that glass of milk, you and that cow are connected. Not only are you drinking its milk, but you also ingesting all of the hormones and antibiotics that the cow was given.

Synthetic hormones, such as recombinant bovine growth hormone (rBGH), are often used in dairy cows to increase milk production. The rBGH can lead to higher rates of udder infections in cows (called mastitis), which in turn increases the need for antibiotics to treat those cows. The antibiotic residues found in milk can contribute to allergic reactions in humans and may even contribute to the growth of antibiotic resistant bacteria.

rBGH isn't legally approved for use in Canada, however, since they are used in dairy cows in the United States, and dairy from the USA is available throughout Canada, Canadians often ingest these hormones, too.

If giving up dairy is not for you, perhaps consider opting for organic milk. At least this way, you will be safe from consuming added growth hormones or antibiotics.

BUT, DON'T I NEED MILK FOR STRONG BONES?

Many scientific studies have been done on the topic of cow's milk consumption and bone health. The findings suggest that not only do we barely absorb the calcium in cow's milk, but it actually contributes to increased calcium loss in our bones. Oh, the irony!

Dairy (especially commercially processed dairy) is extremely acidic to the body and especially to the bones. This means, that when you drink commercially processed dairy, you are not only not absorbing adequate calcium from it, but it is actually stripping calcium away from your bones.

IF I AVOID DAIRY HOW WILL I GET ENOUGH CALCIUM?

Many non-dairy sources of calcium are actually richer in nutrients and better absorbed by the body than cow's milk.

Non-dairy Sources of Calcium

- Green vegetables: chard, kale, spinach, beet greens, collards, broccoli and bok choy
- Nuts and seeds such as sesame seeds, almonds, pumpkin seeds
- Tempeh
- Avocado
- Parsley
- Figs
- Carob
- Beans
- Kelp and kombu

If you choose to avoid dairy on a regular basis, you may also consider taking a daily calcium supplement of between 500 mg to 1,000 mg per day.

WHAT TO LOOK FOR ON PRODUCT LABELS WHEN AVOIDING DAIRY

Dairy is not only found in the milk jug, tub of ice cream or brick of cheese; it is also found in many packaged products, baked goods and other items. When avoiding dairy, make sure to look for the following words on product labels:

- Casein, calcium casein, casein hydrolysate, magnesium casein, potassium casein, rennet casein, sodium casein
- Lactalbumin, lactalbumin phosphate, lactoglobulin, lactose
- Whey, whey hydrolysate

DAIRY CONTAINING FOODS TO AVOID

- Cheese (especially processed cheese)
- Cow's milk
- Sour cream
- Pudding/Ice cream
- Butter, butter flavoring, butter fat
- Margarine

CAN I HAVE ANY DAIRY PRODUCTS AT ALL?

* Those with dairy allergies should avoid dairy completely.

Not all dairy is created equal. Cow dairy found in milk, cream, ice cream, sour cream, and cheese is the dairy we want to avoid. Dairy from goats or sheep, on the other hand, are less allergenic, easier to digest and are often easier to handle by those who are lactose intolerant. Fermented dairy such as yogurt and kefir are easy to digest and actually contain beneficial bacteria that help to promote good bowel health.

Sheep and Goat Milk and Cheese - For some people, consuming goat's or sheep's milk does not contribute to the same negative effects that cow's milk can. Goat's and sheep's milk tends to be more easily digestible and less allergenic than cow's milk, so those who are sensitive may experience no unpleasant symptoms.

Yogurt and Kefir - For some, consuming fermented products such as unsweetened yogurt and kefir does not cause any symptoms of digestive upset. Yogurt is easier to digest than milk, due to the culturing process it undergoes. Enzymes created during the culturing process help to partially digest the casein (milk protein), making it much easier to digest and absorb. Yogurt contains less lactose than milk, and is therefore easier to digest, even by those who are lactose-intolerant, in some cases. Yogurt also contains beneficial bacteria that promote healthy digestion and overall health.

For those with lactose intolerance and/or dairy allergies: Increasing your intake of probiotic-rich foods, as well as taking a high-quality probiotic supplement daily, may help to relieve symptoms associated with lactose intolerance and dairy allergies. *For more on this see page 121.*

But, What Will I Dunk My Cookies In If I Don't Have Milk?

The good news is that avoiding dairy doesn't mean you will be deprived of sporting the perfect white milk mustache, as there are many dairy-free milk alternatives on the market.

DAIRY-FREE MILK ALTERNATIVES

Rice Milk

- Light, sweet tasting milk produced from rice.
- Though commonly unsweetened, rice milk has a naturally sweet taste.
- It is important to choose a whole grain variety of rice milk fortified with vitamins A, D, B12, iron, niacin, and calcium.
- For an extra bit of joy, try chocolate or vanilla flavored rice milk, which is delicious in smoothies, on top of cereal, or right out of the jug.

Almond Milk

- Nutritious, antioxidant rich beverage made from almonds.
- Much like cow's milk, almond milk is a good source of calcium and vitamin D and is also rich in magnesium, iron, zinc, and vitamins.
- Almond milk is not only a substitute for cow's milk but is a healthy option that everyone can enjoy (although those with nut allergies should strictly avoid it).
- Low in calories and free of saturated fat and cholesterol, it is a heart and waist friendly option.

Hemp Milk

- Creamy, nutty tasting milk made from hemp seeds.
- It is a great source of omega-3 and omega-6 fatty acids necessary for proper brain function, as well as calcium, iron, and all ten essential amino acids.
- Choose an organic variety, made with evaporated cane juice or one that is completely sugar-free.

Coconut Milk

- Coconuts are rich in vitamins C, E, B1, B3, B5 and B6 and minerals including iron, selenium, sodium, calcium, magnesium and phosphorous.
- Coconut milk is lactose free.
- Coconuts contain healthy fat that provide the body with energy, rather than being stored in the body as fat.
- The lauric acid found in coconut is converted in the body into monolaurin, known to protect against viruses.
- Choose coconut milk without added sugar or fillers.
- Canned coconut milk is often thicker and better used in recipes than coconut milk sold in jugs. Canned coconut milk is not ideal for drinking as a beverage.
- Coconut milk sold in jugs, in the milk section of the store, is best used as a dairy-free milk alternative and is lighter and sweeter than canned coconut milk.

DAIRY-FREE YOGURT

- Coconut yogurt
- Rice yogurt
- Almond yogurt

DAIRY-FREE ICE CREAM

- Rice ice cream
- Coconut ice cream
- Dairy-free sorbet with no added sugar

Homemade Ice No-Cream

Fruity Sorbet

1.5 cups frozen fruit
   (mangoes or berries work well)
1 cup water or dairy milk alternative
1 tbsp raw honey

* Combine ingredients in blender and blend until creamy. Place in freezer for at least one hour.

Chocolate Banana Cream

1 banana
¼ cup blueberries
½ tbsp. nut or seed butter
½ tbsp. cacao powder
½ tbsp. pure maple syrup

* Combine ingredients in blender and blend until creamy. Place in freezer for at least one hour.

Sweet Coconut Cream

1 cup coconut milk
2 tbsp. dried unsweetened coconut
1 tsp. pure vanilla extract
1-2 tbsp. raw honey or pure maple syrup

* Combine ingredients in blender and blend until creamy. Place in freezer for at least one hour.

DAIRY-FREE CHEESE

- Vegan Cheese slices or shredded cheese.
- Nutritional yeast provides a cheese like flavour to sauces and casseroles.

Homemade Dairy-Free Cheese-Like Alternative

2 cups cashews (pre-soaked in water for about 4 hours)
1 tbsp. lemon juice
½ cup water
½ tsp. sea salt

* Blend all ingredients in a food processor and then cool in the fridge.

SUMMARY

- Making the choice to go completely dairy-free for at least twenty-one days will help to de-gunk your body and improve digestive function.
- Consuming dairy can lead to symptoms such as gas, bloating, diarrhea, abdominal pain, sinus infections, excess mucous production, and acne.
- On a dairy-free diet, avoid milk, cheese, butter, margarine, pudding and ice cream.
- Avoid the words lactose, whey and casein on product labels.
- Sheep and goat's milk are often easier to digest than cow's milk and are a healthier option.
- Yogurt and kefir are fermented milk products, and are often tolerated by those who are sensitive to dairy.
- If going dairy-free long-term does not suit your lifestyle, try opting for organic milk.
- Dairy-free milk alternatives include: rice milk, hemp milk, coconut milk and almond milk. Drink soymilk in moderation.
- Non-dairy sources of calcium include: nuts and seeds, green vegetables, tempeh, parsley, carob, kelp, and avocado.

GUNK-FREE HABIT #7
Make Fat Your Friend

> **HABIT #7 HOW-TO**: Include "good" fats into your diet, while making sure to strictly avoid "bad" fats. Try including a healthy fat at each meal.

I DON'T GET IT – YOU WANT ME TO EAT MORE FAT? I THOUGHT FAT WAS BAD FOR ME.

There is a common misconception that consuming fat will make you fat. And, although it is true that the consumption of saturated and trans fats lead to weight gain, obesity, and even diabetes, the consumption of "good" fats does the exact opposite.

Yes, you heard right, eating fat actually helps us lose fat. We also need fat to reduce inflammation, promote healthy skin, hair, and nails, and for proper brain function. But, we need the right types of fat.

It is important to identify the different types of fat and how they affect our bodies. As part of a healthy, gunk-free diet, we want to avoid all "bad" fats while making sure to consume some of the "good" fats on a regular basis. Roughly twenty-five percent of your daily calorie intake should come from the "good" fats.

It is essential to examine what these "bad" fats are doing to your body and learn why it is so important to incorporate "good" fats into your daily diet.

THE "BAD" FATS

Saturated fats and **trans fats** are known as the "bad" fats. This is because they increase your risk of heart disease, elevate cholesterol levels, lead to weight gain and a host of other diseases.

Unlike the "good" fats, "bad" fats raise our bad cholesterol levels and lower our good cholesterol levels. They also increase our blood pressure.

They increase inflammation in the body, which can be the cause of many life threatening conditions such as strokes, diabetes and heart conditions. Consuming too much bad fat will also result in unhealthy weight gain.

Trans fat are the most dangerous type of fat. Trans fats are found in **hydrogenated or partially hydrogenated oils.** It is extremely important to read the ingredients of every product you choose to make sure you do not see the word "hydrogenated." This word means that the product contains "bad" fats. There is no healthy level of trans fats, and in fact, you should avoid them at all costs. Avoid any food product where the label includes trans fats, as they are extremely harmful to our body. Saturated fats, especially from animal products, should be limited.

"Bad" Fats That We Want to Avoid
- High fat meats (beef, pork)
- Whole fat dairy (cream and milk)
- Cheese (especially processed cheese)
- Ice cream (made with dairy)
- Lard
- Commercially baked pastries, cookies, muffins and cakes
- Packaged snack foods that contain saturated or trans fat (chips, crackers, cookies)
- Margarine
- Vegetable shortening
- Fried foods (French fries, chicken nuggets, or anything breaded or fried)

THE "GOOD" FATS

Monounsaturated and **polyunsaturated** fats are known as the "good" fats. This is because they are good for your heart and overall health. They help to boost metabolism, protect the immune system, and help to reduce inflammation in the body, allowing it to heal properly. They help to balance blood sugar levels and are necessary for the production of hormones in the body.

"Good" Fats to Include in Your Diet

- Flax seeds, chia seeds, sunflower seeds, sesame seeds
- Beans
- Soybeans
- Avocados
- Olive oil
- Coconut oil
- Flax and hemp oils
- Nuts (almonds, hazelnuts, pecans, cashews, walnuts)
- Fatty fish (salmon, tuna, mackerel, herring, sardines, trout, black cod)
    » Consuming fresh fish is recommended. Limit your intake of canned fish, as many contain added sodium and heavy metals.

We've all heard about the omega fats, but what exactly are they and why are they so good for us?

Omega-3 fatty acids are a type of polyunsaturated fat. They are known to help reduce the risk of heart disease, stroke and cancer, help reduce inflammation and promote proper brain function. Omega 3's are considered essential because our bodies do not produce them, and therefore we must obtain them from food.

Fish Oil

The best sources of omega-3 fatty acids are fatty fish such as salmon, herring, mackerel, sardine, trout, black cod, and tuna. These fish contain both EPA (eicosapentaenoic acid) and DHA (docosahexaenoic acid), which are two highly beneficial types of omega-3 fatty acids. Both DHA and EPA are anti-inflammatory. EPA helps to regulate inflammation, blood clotting and circulation, while DHA is necessary for proper brain function and healthy joints.

Fish oil is highly beneficial for preventing and managing cardiovascular disease, diabetes, high blood pressure, osteoporosis, high cholesterol, depression, asthma, arthritis, inflammatory bowel disease and cancer.

It is beneficial to consume at least two to three servings of omega-3 rich fish every week, or a total of six to eight ounces. Consuming fish is one way to meet this recommendation, however, supplementing with fish oil is also beneficial.

When supplementing wish fish oil, make sure to choose one with at least one to two grams total of EPA and DHA together per serving.

Fish-Free Omega-3

Other sources of omega-3 fatty acids include flaxseeds, flax seed oil, walnuts, and soybeans. These items are rich in ALA (alpha linolenic acid). ALA converts into DHA and EPA in the body and helps to reduce inflammation, improve bowel function and promote healthy hair, skin and nails.

Take one to two tablespoons of flax seed oil daily.

Consult your health care provider before supplementing with fish oil or flax seed oil, if you are taking blood-thinning medication.

USING HEALTHY OILS

The following oils are incredibly healthy and can be used on a daily basis. Cold-pressed oils are the best option. These oils are not only tasty, but they provide incredible health benefits.

Oils that can be used for Cooking at High Heat

Although these oils can be used at high heat, they can also be used in a variety of ways that do not involve cooking.

Coconut Oil

- Coconut oil, although a source of saturated fat, contains medium chain fatty acids that provide a quick source of energy and can contribute to weight loss.
- Helps to raise good cholesterol levels and is rich in antioxidants.
- Contains lauric, capric and caprylic acids, which have anti-microbial, anti-bacterial and anti-fungal benefits.
- Coconut oil helps to reduce gas and bloating.

Using Coconut oil

- Coconut oil is very stable and can be used to cook at high temperatures.
- Choose virgin, cold-pressed coconut oil.
- Perfect for baking, roasting, and sautéing, and can even be added to smoothies.
- Can be used as an alternative to butter in baked goods (use 25% less oil than you would if you were using butter).
- Can also be used to moisturize the skin (apply to skin after a bath or shower).
- Coconut oil is solid at room temperature.

Grape Seed Oil

- Grape seed oil is a source of vitamin E, zinc, calcium, phosphorus and magnesium.
- Anti-inflammatory, anti-oxidant, anti-aging, and antimicrobial.
- Beneficial for arthritis, skin conditions, weight loss, high cholesterol, diabetes and protecting the immune system.

Using Grape Seed Oil

- Grape seed oil has a high smoke point, and is therefore able to withstand high temperature cooking.
- Has a light, clean flavour, which makes it suitable for dishes that don't require extra flavour from oil.
- Grape seed oil is a great alternative to vegetable oil.
- Choose cold-pressed grape seed oil stored in glass containers.
- Store in a cool dry place for up to a year.

Oils that can be used for Cooking at Medium Heat

Red Palm Oil

- Red palm oil comes from the fruit of the oil palm tree.
- It is different than regular palm oil, which is heavily processed.

- Has a high concentration of carotenes (antioxidant), which is why it retains a bright red color.
- It is rich in vitamins A and E.
- Contains cholesterol-lowering fatty acids.
- Helps to protect against heart disease.

Using Red Palm Oil

- Has a savory flavour.
- Can be used with fish, stir-fry, oatmeal, in smoothies, or any other healthy dish.
- Choose a virgin, organic red palm oil stored in a glass jar.
- Red palm oil can be used for cooking up to a medium heat.

Avocado Oil

- Rich in vitamins A, D, and E.
- Contains lutein, which helps to reduce aging.
- Helps to protect your cardiovascular system by lowering levels of "bad" cholesterol and triglycerides.

Using Avocado Oil

- Avocado oil has a buttery flavour that helps to enhance the flavour of many dishes.
- Can be used in salad dressing, dips, and smoothies.
- Can be used for cooking up to a medium heat.
- Choose organic, cold-pressed avocado oil stored in an opaque glass bottle.

Olive Oil

- Olive oil contains polyunsaturated and monounsaturated fatty acids.
- Olive oil has been linked to healthier body weight, lower cholesterol, and decreased inflammation.

Using Olive Oil

Choose cold-pressed, extra virgin olive oil stored in a glass bottle.

Can be used for light sautéing or cooking up to a medium heat, in salad dressing, dips, or drizzled over food for flavour.

Oils that Should Not be Heated

It is important to note that **hemp oil and flaxseed oil are extremely susceptible to damage from heat, light, and oxygen.** When exposed to these elements for too long, the oil becomes rancid and loses nutritional value. **Do not cook with these oils,** but instead use them to top salad, drizzle on top of fish or pasta, add to smoothies, etc.

Hemp Oil

- Hemp oil contains the highest percentage of essential omega-3 fatty acids and is made up of 80% polyunsaturated fat ("good" fat).
- Helps to reduce inflammation, protect the heart and promote healthy body weight.

Using Hemp Oil

- Can be added to salad dressing, dips, smoothies, or drizzled over food for flavour.
- Can also be taken on its own as a supplement (1 tbsp. daily) to reduce inflammation, improve hormonal imbalances, and promote healthy hair, skin and nails.
- Hemp oil is not heat stable and therefore should not be used in cooking.
- Choose organic hemp oil stored in a dark bottle.
- Store hemp oil in the fridge to prevent it from going rancid.

Flax Seed Oil

- Flax seed oil is made up of polyunsaturated and monounsaturated fatty acids.
- Flax seed oil provides a source of omega-3 fatty acids, which helps reduce inflammation and promote proper brain function.

Using Flax Seed Oil

- Choose an organic, unrefined brand. Best types are stored in a dark bottle.
- Keep refrigerated in order to prevent rancidity for up to six weeks, or can be frozen for longer.
- Flax seed oil is not heat stable and oxidizes quickly.
- Can be used in salad dressing, dips, smoothies or drizzled over dishes for added flavour.
- Can be taken daily as a supplement (1 tbsp. per day).

SUMMARY

- Include a variety of good fats in your diet, while avoiding bad fats.
- Consume a healthy fat at each meal.
- The "bad" fats are saturated and trans fats. There is no safe level of trans fat and should be avoided completely.
- The "good" fats are polyunsaturated and monounsaturated fats, which help to decrease inflammation, promote proper brain function and support weight loss.
- Consume omega-3 rich foods daily such as, oily fish, flax seeds, soybeans, and walnuts.
- Hemp oil and flax seed oil are incredibly healthful oils. They should not be used at high heat as they are not heat stable. They can be taken daily as a supplement.
- When cooking at high heat, choose grape seed oil or coconut oil.
- When cooking at medium heat, choose red palm oil, avocado oil or olive oil.

GUNK-FREE HABIT #8
Eat Clean Pro-Tein

> **HABIT #8 HOW-TO**: Consume protein at each meal. Limit your intake of red meat to once or twice per week maximum, and always choose lean meats and poultry. Try to have at least one meal each day that is completely vegan (no animal products or dairy). Vegan sources of protein are a great way to meet your daily protein needs. They are lower in fat than animal products, and free of cholesterol.

Protein is an extremely important nutrient that must be obtained in the daily diet. It is crucial for our muscles and is a source of energy for the body. It also helps to stabilize our blood sugar levels, keeping us feeling satisfied and full throughout the day – a great way to curb cravings for sweets. Protein provides us with the essential amino acids that our bodies need in order to function optimally. It is recommended to consume protein at each meal and with each snack.

GUNK-FREE SOURCES OF PROTEIN

Animal-based protein

- Lean meats
- Fish
- Poultry
- Eggs
- High quality New Zealand whey protein powders

Vegan sources (not just for vegans!)

- Legumes
- Nuts and seeds (and butters made from these)
- Tempeh (fermented soy)
- Sprouted tofu
- Green vegetables
- Vegan protein powders

Ideally, we should be consuming **0.8 grams of protein per kilogram of body weight** each day. Consuming adequate protein is extremely important, but choosing the right *types* of protein is equally as imperative. To start, don't worry so much about the exact quantity, but rather focus more on the quality.

Consuming too much animal protein is not recommended. Red meat, chicken and other animal proteins are high in saturated fat and contribute to high cholesterol, weight gain and even diabetes. Consuming these foods in moderation is key. Even white meat chicken without the skin contains significant amounts of "bad" fat. About twenty-three percent of the calories in a breast of chicken come from fat, and much of that is saturated fat. This increases cholesterol and worsens insulin resistance, which can contribute to diabetes.

When choosing your animal protein, it is best to choose organic, grass-fed, free-range meats. This means that the animals have been raised in healthy, open conditions and have not been fed grains or given antibiotics or hormones. Look for words such as "no added hormones" or "from cows not treated with rBGH".

Organic or free-range eggs are another protein-rich food, which can be consumed as part of a gunk-free diet. When consuming fish, choose wild-caught fish as much as possible.

> **Gunk-Free Tip:**
> Instead of using eggs in cooking or baking (for a vegan, allergy-friendly option):
> - Combine 1 tbsp. chia seeds with 3 tbsp. warm water and let stand until it forms a gelatinous solution. This replaces one egg.
> - Combine 1 tbsp. ground flax seeds with 3 tbsp. water and let stand. This replaces one egg.
> - ¼ cup applesauce or 1 banana can also be used to replace one egg.

GUNK-FILLED PROTEIN TO AVOID

- Processed deli meat (corned beef, pastrami, ham, turkey, bologna and others).
- Bacon, sausage, hot dogs.
- Red meat – in large amounts (limit to once or twice per week maximum)
- Processed soy - soymilk, tofu (unless it is sprouted), soy burgers, soy hot dogs.
- Protein powders made with refined sugar, artificial sweeteners, added fillers and other artificial ingredients.

THE SOY STORY

Soy is commonly consumed as an animal-free, vegan protein option. However, just because soy doesn't come from a cow, doesn't mean that it is the best option. Soy has been linked to malnutrition, digestive distress, thyroid dysfunction, reproductive disorders and infertility. Soy contains goitrogens, which block the synthesis of thyroid hormones in the body, therefore affecting thyroid function. It also contains isoflavones, which are a type of phytoestrogen. These phytoestrogens resemble human estrogen and can mimic and even block estrogen in the body, causing disruption to proper endocrine function, infertility and may even lead to breast cancer.

Phytic acid in soy hinders the absorption of some nutrients in the body. It is heavily processed and heavily sprayed with pesticides, and is genetically modified in most cases. Phytoestrogens in soy lead to early development and puberty, as well as decrease testosterone levels. It is also important to avoid feeding your child soymilk or soy formula.

Gunk-Filled Soy to Avoid

- Tofu
- Soybean oil
- Soymilk

- Soy cheese and soy yogurt
- Soy meat (meatless burgers and hot dogs)

Soy is used in many packaged foods, so make sure to read food labels and watch out for added soy.

Not all soy is created equal...

Fermented soy products like miso, tempeh, natto, organic soybeans and soy sauces (wheat-free, such as Tamari) are good for us and can be consumed regularly. Fermenting creates probiotic qualities, which helps digestion and stops the process of phytic acid. Fermentation occurs when no oxygen is present and at low temperatures.

More about tempeh and miso on pages 122-123.

SHAKE UP YOUR PROTEIN

Protein shakes are a great way to start the day. They are also great as a snack or before/after a workout. A protein shake is a great way to ensure that you are getting all of essential amino acids that your body requires on a regular basis, since it can be difficult to meet our daily protein needs on food alone (especially for those who do not consume animal products). Drinking a high quality protein shake allows for easy and quick absorption into the body, as the body does not have to do much work to break it down – much less than it would have to for steak, chicken, or fish.

Protein in liquid form, as oppose to food, is much easier on the body and provides quick energy and nourishment. Food sources can take up to two hours to process, whereas a protein shake takes only thirty minutes.

Consume a high quality protein powder, mixed with fresh fruits, vegetables and perhaps even some superfoods (see page 101). Adding healthy ingredients to your protein shake helps to increase energy, increase mood, improve digestion, aid with weight loss and contribute to overall good health.

CHOOSING A PROTEIN POWDER

Non-dairy (vegan) protein powders are often easier to digest than whey protein, and contribute to less inflammation and mucus production in the body – thus, less gunk. Vegan protein powders are often made from brown rice, hemp, and pea proteins. They provide a good source of protein and energy without causing digestive upset. They are perfect for those who are sensitive or who simply choose to avoid dairy.

Vegan Protein Powders

- It is beneficial to choose a raw, sprouted vegan protein powder as this helps with digestibility.
- Choose a brand with no added sugar, fillers, artificial flavours or colors.

Whey Protein Powders

Whey protein has the highest biological value of any protein. It is suitable for those who choose to consume dairy, however, those who are sensitive or allergic to dairy should avoid it.

- It is essential to choose a whey protein made with whey protein isolate or a blend of whey isolate and concentrate.
- Choose New Zealand whey. New Zealand whey is the cleanest, purest form of whey available. The New Zealand dairy industry has incredibly high standards for product safety and the humane treatment of their cows. Their cows are never injected with growth hormones, antibiotics, genetically modified organisms, or any other chemicals. The cows graze in grass pastures, where the air is clean and the water is fresh.
- Choosing a brand with added enzymes such as protease, lactase and amylase is recommended, as these enzymes help to make the protein more digestible.
- Choose one that is hormone and antibiotic free.
- Choose an all-natural brand, free of refined sugars, artificial flavours and artificial colors.
- Choose one that is GMO-free.

More smoothie recipes on pages 180-182.

SUMMARY

- Consume protein at each meal and each snacks – lean meats, fish, poultry, eggs, protein powder, legumes, nuts and seeds, tempeh, sprouted tofu and green vegetables.
- Limit your intake of red meat to once or twice per week maximum.
- Try to have one meal each day that is completely vegan (no animal products or dairy).
- When choosing animal protein, choose organic, grass fed, free-range meats and organic, free-range eggs.
- When choosing fish, choose wild-caught as much as possible.
- Avoid deli meat, bacon, sausage, hot dogs, and processed soy.
- Protein shakes are an easily digestible and absorbable way to meet your daily protein needs.

GUNK-FREE HABIT #9
Time to Veg

> **HABIT #9 HOW-TO**: Consume a variety of colorful fruits and vegetables. Incorporate seven to ten servings of fruits and vegetables into your daily diet. Try to incorporate leafy green vegetables into each meal.

A serving of fresh or frozen vegetables is ½ cup, and a serving of leafy green vegetables is 1 cup. A serving of fresh or frozen fruit is ½ cup or 1 medium sized fruit.

It is easy to get stuck on eating the same types of fruits and vegetables each day (like carrots and apples), and neglect the amazing variety of nutrient-packed fruits and vegetables available. Consuming any fresh produce is a great start, but the big goal is to incorporate between seven to ten servings of fruits and vegetables into your diet each day. It's also about making sure that you are getting your leafy greens in.

If you are not used to consuming seven to ten servings of fruits and vegetables each day, it can seem overwhelming. The trick is to take it slowly and work your way up. Start by including one serving of vegetables at each meal and perhaps one fruit as part of a snack. Eventually, you will notice that meeting your daily needs is quite simple and painless.

The key is to consume more vegetables than fruit, as fruit contains more sugar than vegetables. Consuming approximately two to three servings of fruit per day is recommended.

FRUITS AND VEGETABLES

Colorful fruits and vegetables provide our bodies with vitamins, minerals, enzymes, and phytonutrients. Many are rich in fiber, which helps to promote proper bowel function, thus reducing symptoms of constipation and/or diarrhea. They also help to reduce inflammation in the body, decrease cholesterol levels, and protect our eyes and vision.

Some Nutrient Packed Fruits and Vegetables

- **Carrots** - High in beta-carotene and antioxidants.
- **Celery** - A good source of natural sodium. Promotes tissue flexibility.
- **Beets** – Powerful for detoxifying the liver and purifying the blood.
- **Cabbage**- High in vitamin C, helps to protect and enhance our immune system.
- **Apples** - High in vitamin C, Vitamin A and antioxidants. Also great for flushing out the liver and has anti-carcinogenic properties.
- **Spinach** – Provides a large dose of iron and chlorophyll.
- **Blackberries** – A powerful antioxidant. Also high in vitamin C, folic acid and potassium.
- **Kale** – Rich in iron and calcium. Great for detoxifying the body and is packed with antioxidants.
- **Pineapple** – Contains bromelain – a natural digestive enzyme that helps to break down the foods we eat. It is anti-inflammatory and rich in vitamin C.
- **Cucumber** – Rich in potassium and antioxidants. Act as a mild diuretic, which helps with high blood pressure and prevents weight gain.

TIPS FOR ADDING MORE FRUITS AND VEGETABLES TO YOUR DIET

- Include a salad at each meal.
- Add fresh vegetables to your favourite sandwich.
- Snack on vegetables throughout the day – cut up some celery, carrot and cucumber and serve with your favourite dip. ***Dip recipes on pages 182-183.***
- Make a smoothie – the easiest way to meet your daily fruit and vegetable needs is to toss them into a smoothie. Try adding kale or spinach to your favorite smoothie. You don't taste the vegetables, but you do retain all of the nutrients from them. ***Smoothie recipes pages 180-182.***

- Add vegetables to homemade stir-fry, casseroles, pasta, and pizza.
- Consume apple or pear slices with your favourite nut or seed butter as part of a healthy snack.
- Add fresh berries to your morning oatmeal or yogurt.
- Add leafy green vegetables to your favourite soup recipe.
- Add leafy green vegetables to omelets.

FRUITS TO CONSUME MORE OF

- Berries – blueberry, strawberry, blackberry, raspberry
- Apple
- Pear
- Peach
- Mango
- Banana
- Cherry
- Orange
- Lime
- Lemon
- Plum
- Kiwi
- Papaya
- Pineapple
- Any fresh fruit that does not cause a reaction.

Those with high blood sugar or diabetes should avoid fruit with a high glycemic index including, bananas, watermelon and pineapple.

Taking Medication? Say NO to Grapefruit!

If taking medication, avoid grapefruit, as it can interfere with the medication and can be fatal. Grapefruit contains a chemical compound, which blocks the enzyme that normally breaks down certain medications in the body. Overtime, the medication levels build up in the body and can become toxic.

There are a number of drugs that may interact with grapefruit, including cholesterol lowering medications, antibiotics, cancer drugs and heart drugs. Speak to your health care provider before consuming grapefruit if you are taking medication of any kind.

VEGETABLES TO CONSUME MORE OF

- Asparagus
- Cucumber
- Celery
- Carrots
- Leek
- Mushrooms
- Beets
- Onion
- Bell peppers
- Tomatoes
- Zucchini
- Sweet potato
- Yam
- Turnip
- Cruciferous vegetables including
  » Broccoli
  » Cauliflower
  » Cabbage
  » Radish
  » Brussels sprouts

LEAFY GREEN VEGETABLES

- Spinach
- Kale
- Bok choy
- Mustard greens
- Collard greens
- Swiss chard
- Rapine
- Dandelion greens
- Arugula
- Watercress
- Beet greens

Why We Need Leafy Greens

Dark leafy green vegetables are one of the most concentrated sources of nutrients found in any food. They are rich sources of minerals, including iron, calcium, potassium, and magnesium, as well as vitamins, including vitamins K, C, E, and many of the B vitamins.

Green vegetables are rich in antioxidants, help to promote proper digestion, help to alkalinize the body as well as promote detoxification. Aside from being nutritional powerhouses, the vegetables are also extremely low in calories and high in fiber.

Using Leafy Greens

When consuming these green veggies, it is best to eat them raw or lightly steamed, as this retains the highest nutrient content.

They can also be added to soups, stews and salads or blended into your favourite smoothie recipe. Making a fresh green juice in the morning is also beneficial. Leafy green veggies should be consumed every single day as part of a healthy diet.

Always make sure to wash you leafy green vegetables well and remove the stems before consuming.

> **Gunk-Free Tip**: Wash celery and place stalks it into a glass jar, container, or bowl filled with cold water. Place into fridge for up to ten days, changing the water every two to three days. The water helps to keep the celery fresh and crunchy, and prevents wilting.

DELICIOUS GREEN VEGGIE RECIPES

Kale Chips

- Preheat an oven to 350°F.
- With a knife or kitchen shears remove the leaves from the thick stems of kale and tear into bite size pieces.
- Wash and thoroughly dry kale.
- Drizzle kale with olive oil (about 1 tbsp.) and sprinkle with sea salt.
- Bake (on a baking sheet) for approximately 10-12 minutes, until crispy.
- Enjoy!

* If you have a little more time to spare - Preheat your oven to 200°F and bake for two hours until crispy.

Green Juice

- 1 apple
- 1 handful parsley
- 2 stalks celery
- 2 cups spinach
- 1 cup dandelion greens
- ½ large cucumber
- ½ lemon

* Juice items in a juicer or blender. See instructions for blender juicing on page 98.

Sesame and Garlic Spinach

Ingredients

- 3 tbsp. dark sesame oil
- 1 tbsp. minced garlic
- 1 lb. fresh spinach - remove large stems and discard, roughly chop the leaves
- 1 tbsp. soy sauce (Braggs or Tamari)
- Sea salt to taste
- 1 tbsp. toasted sesame seeds

Instructions

- Toast sesame seeds – add 1 tsp. grape seed oil to skillet on medium heat. Add sesame seeds, stirring constantly until they begin to brown. Place in a bowl.
- Heat 2 tbsp. of sesame oil in large skillet over medium heat. Add garlic and sauté for 2-3 minutes. Add spinach and cook until it begins to wilt. Turn heat to low.

- Add soy sauce and remove from heat.
- Add sea salt to taste.
- Sprinkle with toasted sesame seeds.

Kale and Cabbage Coleslaw

Ingredients

1 bunch of kale – in small pieces

1 bunch of swiss chard – in small pieces

1 head of cabbage (purple) - shredded

1 beet – shredded

2 tbsp sesame seeds

Dressing ingredients

¼ cup flaxseed oil

½ cup apple cider vinegar

½ lemon, freshly squeezed

pinch of sea salt

1 tbsp. honey

Instructions

- Shred cabbage and beets
- Tear kale and chard into small pieces
- In a large bowl, mix all ingredients together (except for sesame seeds)
- Add dressing
- Mix by hand and massage lightly to soften the kale and Swiss chard
- Refrigerate for 30 minutes
- Add sesame seeds before serving

SUMMARY

- Consume a variety of fruits and vegetables daily (try to incorporate them at each meal).
- Aim for roughly 7-10 servings of fresh fruits and vegetables per day. Choose colorful ones.
- Do not consume grapefruit if you are taking medication. This can have serious and even fatal side effects.
- Include leafy green vegetables into your diet. Eat them raw or lightly steamed. Eat them every day.

GUNK-FREE HABIT #10
Drink Water, Water and More Water

> **HABIT #10 HOW-TO**: Drink at least eight glasses of fresh, pure, clean water everyday. This is one of the best ways to detoxify our bodies, speed up metabolism, and prevent dehydration.

Water is so incredibly important to the human body and to our health. Two thirds of our bodies are made up of water, and without it, we would not survive. Drinking water is such a simple practice, and yet most people do not drink enough of it on a daily basis. It is VITAL for you to increase your water intake (if you are not already drinking at least eight glasses per day) to ensure that you are adequately hydrated, and to promote proper detoxification and elimination.

WHY WE NEED WATER

All of the cells and organs that make up our bodies need water for proper functioning. Water is responsible for transporting nutrients and oxygen into our cells. It also acts as a lubricant and protects our muscle and joints. Water is extremely important for proper digestion as well. Not only does it work together with fiber to help regulate bowel movements, but insufficient water intake can actually slow down your metabolism. Without water, the liver cannot metabolize fat into useable energy, and improper water intake can lead to weight gain. Water also serves as a natural detoxifier, by helping to flush out toxins that are harmful to our bodies. It helps to support the immune system, as well as helps to reduce inflammation.

Water also serves as a natural remedy for headache or back pain, and also ensures that skin stays healthy, fresh and youthful. Water helps to replenish skin tissues, moisturizes skin and increases skin elasticity. All in all, proper hydration brings about good health and wellness.

Water helps to oxygenate the brain and helps to promote focus and alertness. It helps to reduce mid-day brain-fog.

Our bodies lose water on a daily basis through breathing, sweating, urine and bowel movements. Therefore, it is essential to replenish this water loss. Factors such as lifestyle, level of exercise, health status, and climate determine our daily water needs.

- **Lifestyle** – alcohol and caffeine consumption require an additional consumption of two cups of water per alcoholic or caffeinated beverage.
- **Exercise** – we lose water when we sweat, so make sure to consume adequate water when exercising.
- **Environment** – hot and humid weather requires extra intake of fluid.
- **Health** – fever, diarrhea, and vomiting all contribute to additional loss of body fluids, which must be replenished.
- **Pregnant and breast-feeding women** - expecting mothers and those who are breast-feeding require additional fluid intake in order to stay hydrated.

WATER AND WEIGHT LOSS

Water can act as an appetite suppressant. **Drink one glass of cold water about thirty minutes to one hour before each meal to curb appetite and prevent over eating.** Cold water takes time to warm up to body temperature when consumed, and is therefore not absorbed in the body as quickly as room temperature water. This provides a feeling of fullness and helps to curb cravings and prevent overeating.

SOURCES OF WATER

Not all water properly serves the body. The quality of the water that we drink is equally as important as the quantity.

Water to Avoid (as much as possible)

It is important to avoid tap water, distilled water, and deionized water as much as possible. All of these sources have been put through processes that strip the water of its essential minerals. It is important to avoid any water that has been treated with chlorine or has high levels of fluoride. Tap water, for example, can contain contaminants such as organic material, excreted medications, hormones and fluoride. It is also often treated with chlorine in order to kill bacteria and other contaminants. Chlorine does a good job of destroying pathogens in our water, but it also contributes to unbalanced digestive tract flora and poor health.

It is also important to avoid "vitamin water", as most are filled with high fructose corn syrup, artificial colors, preservatives and caffeine. Carbonated water should also be avoided, as it can contribute to gas, bloating and digestive upset.

It is recommended to avoid plastic bottled water. There are dangerous chemicals and toxins in the plastic of these bottles that leach into the water. Not only is avoiding bottled water better for our health, but it is also much better for the environment. If bottled water is something that you choose to purchase, make sure the plastic bottles are free of BPA (this chemical is hazardous to our health).

Water to Drink

Good sources of water include natural spring water, filtered water, artesian water, reverse-osmosis, or mineral water from an underground source. Using a carbon filter at home is practical and cost effective, however, it does not completely filter out all unwanted particles. That being said, any filter is better than no filter at all. Use a stainless steel or BPA-free bottle for your water, or purchase water that is stored in glass bottles.

> **Gunk-Free Tip**: Do not drink water with your meals as this will dilute your stomach acid and prevent your food from breaking down properly. Small sips are fine. In addition, wait at least 30-45 minutes after eating before drinking water.

SUMMARY

- Drink at least eight glasses of fresh, pure, clean water everyday.
- Drink one glass of cold water about thirty minutes to one hour before each meal to curb appetite and prevent overeating.
- Avoid tap water, distilled water and deionized water.
- Avoid plastic bottled water. Instead choose glass bottles or use BPA-free or stainless steel bottles.
- Good sources of water include natural spring water, filtered water, artesian water, reverse-osmosis water or mineral water.
- Avoid drinking too much with meals as this dilutes stomach acid and prevents food from being properly broken down.

GUNK-FREE HABIT #11
Squeeze Some Lemon

> **HABIT #11 HOW-TO:** Add the juice of half a fresh lemon to a glass of room temperature or warm water each morning (on an empty stomach before breakfast).

Getting into the habit of starting your day with a glass of lemon water is the simplest but most effective practices you will implement into your daily routine. Lemon water helps to refresh our bodies, detoxify our organs, and improve digestion. It also helps to give our metabolisms a bit of a boost.

WHY ARE LEMONS SO GOOD FOR US?

Lemons Help to Improve Immunity
- Lemons are high in vitamin C, which is great for fighting off colds and infections.
- Helps to keep the body hydrated and helps with congestion.

Lemons Help to Alkalinize
- Although lemons taste acidic, they actually help to alkalinize the body. This helps to keep our internal pH levels balanced, as well as prevents infection and disease.

Lemons Increase Energy and Improve Mood
- Good source of vitamin C, which is one of the first things depleted when the mind and body are exposed to stress.
- Contains brain-protecting flavonoids.
- The scent of lemon has natural mood enhancing properties.

Lemons Promote Detoxification
- Lemons help to clear toxins out of your body, and in turn, will help to make your skin look radiant.
- Help to produce the bile necessary for proper digestion and assimilation.
- Lemons help the liver get rid of free radicals in the body.

- The vitamin C found in lemons aids in the production of glutathione - a key antioxidant that the liver needs for detoxification.

Lemons Improve Digestion

Lemon water is great for relieving digestive upset such as nausea, heartburn, bloating and gas. It is great as a post-meal digestive aid.

Boosts a lethargic appetite and allows for a better flow of digestive juices.

Helps to boost metabolism and aids in the absorption of nutrients.

WHAT ELSE CAN WE DO WITH LEMONS?

Preserve Food

Cut an apple or avocado in half and squeeze some lemon on top to keep it from browning so quickly.

Zesty Lemon Dressing

¼ cup olive oil or flaxseed oil
2-3 tbsp apple cider vinegar (raw, unpasteurized)
½ fresh squeezed lemon
1 tbsp raw honey
pinch of sea salt and pepper to taste
* Mix all ingredients together in bowl

Refreshingly Soothing Lemonade

1 cup freshly squeezed lemon juice
6 cups filtered water
½ cup raw honey
¼ cup aloe juice
Using a lemon juicer or your hands, juice the lemons and pour into a glass jug. Add honey, aloe vera juice and water (can use less water if you like it a bit tangier). Serve cold and store in fridge.

Lemon and Apple Cider Vinegar Detox Drink

This powerful drink works wonders for detoxifying the body, promoting weight loss, improving digestion, and promoting overall better health. Consume on an empty stomach daily, or here and there as you see fit.

Apple cider vinegar is loaded with enzymes and beneficial bacteria. It can help lower blood pressure and balance blood sugar. It helps to increase your body's metabolic rate, allowing you to burn calories more efficiently.

Cayenne helps to speed up metabolism and lower blood pressure. It also helps to clean fat out of the arteries.

> 1 glass of water (12 oz.)
> 2 tbsp. fresh squeezed lemon juice
> 2 tbsp. apple cider vinegar
> ¼ tsp. cayenne pepper
> 1 tsp. pure maple syrup or other natural sweetener (optional)
>
> * Mix all ingredients together in a glass and consume on an empty stomach.

SUMMARY

- Start your day with a glass of lemon water – squeeze half of a fresh lemon into a glass of room temperature or warm water.
- Lemons help to improve immunity, increase energy, alkalinize the body, promote detoxification and improve digestion.
- The lemon and apple cider vinegar detox drink can be consumed daily, or on occasion, in order to promote cleansing and detoxification of the body.

GUNK-FREE HABIT #12
Choose Box-Free Juice

> **HABIT #12 HOW-TO**: Incorporate a fresh, homemade vegetable/fruit juice into your daily diet. Consume on an empty stomach if possible. Best to have in the morning before breakfast. Juice three vegetables for every one fruit. Avoid sugar-filled, concentrated, store-bought juices.

WHAT IS JUICING ALL ABOUT?

Juicing (removing the fiber from fresh fruits and vegetables, and consuming the fresh juice) is one of the most effective ways to cut down on cravings for unhealthy and unnecessary foods. It is the easiest form of food to digest, containing vitamins, alkaline minerals, and enzymes in liquid form. The body immediately assimilates nutrients from the fresh juice, due to its highly absorbable liquid state. This leaves the digestive system with little work to do. Juicing helps to clear the mind, clears skin, detoxifies, and aids with weight loss.

The juices that we want to include in our diet are raw and freshly made, using a juicer or blender. Juices that are found in grocery stores are usually filled with added preservatives and sugars, and contain little to no vitamins and minerals. If you are going to purchase premade juices, ensure that there are no added fillers or sugars and that the juice is dated to expire within a few days from purchase. A short shelf life means that the juice contains fresh ingredients, and that no fillers or preservatives have been added to sustain its life. Fresh juices made right before your eyes are another good option, however, even with these, it is essential to know exactly what is being added to your juice.

When juices are made fresh, daily, the nutrients stay intact, and the enzymes that help us digest our food are retained. Making a healthy and nutritious juice requires extracting all of the liquid from the fresh fruits or vegetables. When you juice, the fiber is eliminated, and all that is left is the liquid, which contains all of the beneficial nutrients. Without the fiber present (which actually slows down the rate of absorption), nutrients go directly to feed our cells.

JUICING FOR WEIGHT LOSS AND DETOXIFICATION

The nutrients provided by juicing fresh, raw fruits and vegetables help to flush out toxins in the body, and at the same time, help to shed weight. Excess toxins in the body can contribute to headaches, infections, lack of energy, depression, weight gain and other severe illnesses. Juicing help to break down these toxins and eliminate them from our systems.

Fresh fruits and vegetables naturally contain enzymes that help to break down our food. Juicing provides us with loads of these digestive enzymes, which helps to reduce digestive upset, promote proper breakdown of food, and therefore helps to flush out and regulate the digestive system, keeping it healthy.

JUICING HELPS TO ALKALINIZE

Getting into the habit of juicing daily will help alkalinize the body and balance your pH levels. This helps to keep your blood healthy and prevents disease. Consuming fresh fruits and vegetables is one of the best ways to alkalinize the body. The benefit of juicing these items is that you can pack multiple servings of fruits and vegetables into one juice.

EQUIPMENT NEEDED FOR JUICING

Juicer

Making a fresh juice everyday does not have to be complicated or expensive. There are a variety of different juicers on the market, so the key is to find one that suits your needs and budget.

Blender

If you do not have a juicer at home, and do not want to purchase one, you can use a blender instead. To juice with a blender, simply add water and your produce to the blender, little by little. There should be enough water to cover all of the produce. Blend until you have sufficient juice. Then, place a glass underneath a strainer or nut milk bag, strain and enjoy!

FOODS TO INCLUDE IN YOUR JUICE

Many fruits and vegetables contain high quality, beneficial nutrients and produce sufficient liquid when juiced. Try some of the following in your juice, or feel free to try any and all fresh vegetables and fruit you like. Get creative and experiment to see what combinations suit your taste.

Remember: Juice three vegetables for every one fruit. Fruits are naturally high in sugar, so it is important to juice vegetables along with your fruit.

Some Suggested Juice Combinations

Green Juice

- ½ large cucumber
- 3-4 kale leaves
- Handful of spinach
- 3 stalks of celery
- ½ lemon
- ½ inch piece of fresh ginger

Digestive Juice

- ½ pineapple (peeled)
- 2 stalks celery
- ½ large cucumber
- 2 handfuls spinach

Love your Liver

4 large carrots
4 stalks of celery
1 handful of dandelion greens or 1 handful of kale
½ apple

V-7 Juice

2 tomatoes
1 bunch parsley
2 medium carrots
4 stalks of celery
3 handfuls spinach
½ beet
½ head romaine lettuce
pinch of cayenne
pinch sea salt

Sweet Beet

1 stalk celery
1 carrot
½ orange
½ lemon
1 beet
2 handfuls spinach

Add some wheatgrass, chlorophyll or spirulina powder to any juice for some added detoxifying action.

SUMMARY

- Incorporate a fresh vegetable/fruit juice into your daily diet. Consume on an empty stomach.
- Fresh juice is the easiest form of food to digest and provides the body with immediate nourishment.
- Juice three vegetables for every one fruit.

GUNK-FREE HABIT #13
Say Yes to Superfoods

> **HABIT #13 HOW-TO:** Include at least one superfood into your daily diet. These nutrient packed superfoods will leave you feeling nourished, energized, and detoxified.

SUPERFOODS? DO THEY HAVE SUPER POWERS OR SOMETHING?

The answer is, yes! Superfoods are really just what they sound like – super foods. Their nutritional content is so powerful and their benefits are so incredible that they have been categorized into their own class of foods. They contain vitamins, minerals, and other nutrients that help to prevent disease and promote overall health and vitality.

Superfoods contain high concentrations of various antioxidants, anthocyanins, vitamin C, manganese, and dietary fiber. They help to improve energy, promote weight loss, reduce inflammation, promote detoxification, and a long list of other health benefits.

There are a wide variety of superfoods to choose from. You don't always have to stick to the same one or two, and feel free to include as many of these foods into your daily diet as you like.

CHIA SEEDS

- Chia seeds are tiny little seeds that come from the Salvia hispanica plant, a member of the mint family.
- Chia seeds help to balance blood sugar and prevent food cravings – therefore they are great for diabetics.
- They turn into a gel like substance in the body (or when mixed with a liquid). They expand and bulk up, keeping us feeling full for longer.
- Chia seeds provide long lasting energy.

- Great source of fiber, which helps with constipation and proper elimination.
- Good source of omega-3 fatty acids, which are needed for proper brain function, as well as healthy hair, skin and nails.
- Help to reduce inflammation and lower cholesterol.
- A complete protein that provides us with all of the amino acids that our bodies need.

3.5 ounces of chia seeds is equivalent to consuming:

- 10 ounces of spinach for iron
- 23 ounces of milk for calcium
- 6 ounces of bananas for potassium
- 53 ounces of broccoli for magnesium

Using Chia Seeds

- Add 1-2 tbsp. of chia seeds to smoothies, salads, yogurt, oatmeal, desserts, on toast with nut or seed butter, dips, jams or puddings.

Chia can be used to replace eggs in cooking or baking for a vegan friendly, low cholesterol recipe.

- To replace one egg in a recipe - Mix 1 tablespoons of ground chia seeds with 3 tbsp. water. Let it sit for 5-10 minutes.

Ch-Ch-Ch-Chocolate Chia Pudding

Ingredients

1 cup milk alternative (almond milk, hemp milk, rice milk, coconut milk)
1 tbsp. pure maple syrup or raw honey
1 tsp. cocoa powder or cacao powder
2 tbsp. chia seeds
½ tsp. pure vanilla extract
2 tbsp. unsweetened coconut (optional)
¼ cup fresh berries (optional)

Preparation

- Place milk alternative, maple syrup or honey, cocoa powder, vanilla, and chia seeds into blender, and blend until it begins to thicken.
- Place into bowl and refrigerate for ½ hour (at least), until chilled. It will thicken the longer it remains in the fridge.
- Remove from fridge and top with fresh berries and/or coconut (or other topping of choice).

Raspberry Chia Jam

Ingredients

1.5 cups frozen or fresh raspberries
1 tbsp. fresh squeezed lemon juice
2 tbsp. water
2 tbsp. raw honey or pure maple syrup
3 tbsp. chia seeds

Preparation

* If using frozen raspberries, allow them to thaw to room temperature

- Place raspberries in a bowl and crush them using a fork.
- Add lemon juice, water, honey/maple syrup, and chia seeds.
- Pour mixture into jar with lid.
- Refrigerate for at least one hour. You will notice it thicken with time.

* Can be eaten right from the jar, on toast with nut or seed butter, with crackers, on top of chicken, or anyway you like.

FLAX SEEDS

- Flax seeds are powerful seeds that come from the flax plant.
- They are completely gluten-free and loaded with fiber.
- They help to promote proper bowel function.

- They contain large amounts of polyunsaturated oil, which is high in omega-3 and omega-6 fatty acids.
- The omega content of flax seeds help to reduce the risk of heart disease and cancer, and help to raise our levels of good cholesterol.
- Helps to decrease inflammation, including inflammation in the arteries, which may help to prevent heart attacks and stroke.

Using Flax Seeds

- Add 1-2 tbsp. of ground flax seeds to your favourite smoothie, on top of oatmeal, or sprinkle into your salad dressing.
- Flax seeds must be ground in order for us to digest and absorb them. They can be purchased whole (which requires grinding) or ground (which must be kept refrigerated).

Ground versus Whole Flax

Ground flax seeds provide more nutritional benefits than whole seeds. Whole seeds have a tough outer layer, which prevents the seeds from being broken down in the digestive system. Whole flax seeds go through our bodies whole, and end up just coming out the other end without being digested – a nutrient-rich poop is all that you are left with.

The oil in flax is highly unsaturated, which means that it oxidizes and goes rancid quickly once the seed is ground. Whole flax has a tough outer shell that protects it from oxidation. When the seed is broken or ground, the volatile oils are released, and rancidity can occur. This is why they must be kept refrigerated.

Buying whole flax seeds

Purchasing whole flax seeds means that you will need to grind them yourself using a coffee grinder, food processor or blender. Once ground, they must be stored in the fridge or freezer. The benefit of buying whole flax seeds is that they have a longer shelf life than ground seeds. You can grind them as you need them, or grind a small batch and keep them in the fridge for daily use. Whole flax seeds should be stored in a cool, dry, dark place. Although not essential, storing them in the fridge helps to ensure freshness.

Buying ground flax seeds

Always keep ground flax seeds in an airtight container in the fridge. Once the seeds are ground, they are more susceptible to becoming rancid. In order to prevent rancidity, store them in the fridge for up to ninety days. You can also freeze them, which helps to keep them fresher longer.

Is there a difference between brown and yellow flax seeds?

The only real difference between brown and yellow flax is their color. They are both rich in fiber, omega-3 fatty acids, and lignans. So, choose your color freely.

HEMP SEEDS

- Hemp is a complete vegetarian source of protein (great for both vegetarians and non-vegetarians).
- Provides the ideal ratio of omega-6 to omega-3 fatty acids. (The World Health Organization recommends a 4:1 ratio, and hemp provides a ratio of 3.71:1).
- Helps to support heart health, reduce inflammation and balance hormones.
- Rich in fiber and helps to promote proper bowel function.
- Helps to facilitate fat burning due to its GLA (gamma linolenic acid) content.
- Rich in zinc, calcium, magnesium and iron.

Using Hemp Seeds

Add 1-2 tbsp. of hemp seeds to your favourite smoothie, on top of oatmeal, or sprinkle into your salad dressing.

CACAO

Cacao is raw, naturally sugar-free, pure chocolate. All of the bad things commonly attributed to chocolate bars, such as cavities, weight gain and diabetes, are actually caused by the dairy, sugar, and other fillers added to the dark chocolate, and not necessarily the chocolate itself.

Benefits of Cacao

- Rich in antioxidants and magnesium, which help to balance brain chemistry and build strong bones.
- Helps to boost serotonin levels, which keeps us feeling happy.
- Increases focus and alertness.

The Difference Between Cacao and Cocoa

Cacao: Refers to the tree, its pods, and the beans inside.

Cocoa: Refers to two by-products of the cacao bean – cocoa powder and cocoa butter. Both are extracted from the bean when it is processed in the factory.

Using Cacao

- Add raw cacao nibs or cacao powder to smoothies, dessert recipes, or eat the nibs right out of the bag! Cacao is not sweet. Do not use to sweeten food.

SPIRULINA

- Spirulina is named for its spiral shape and belongs to the family of cyanobacteria or blue-green microalgae.
- It's the highest protein food - over sixty percent all-digestible vegetable protein, which is even more than cooked steak, which consists of only twenty-five percent protein.
- It has the highest concentration of beta-carotene, vitamin B-12, and iron than any other food.
- Helps to alkalinize and detoxify the body.
- Boosts energy levels and improves concentration.

- Helps to control blood sugar levels and cravings, which makes it highly beneficial for diabetics and those wanting to lose weight.

Using Spirulina

- Start with one gram of spirulina powder per day (1/4 tsp) mixed in water, juice, or a smoothie during the first week.
- Increase the dose gradually over the following weeks to between two to five grams daily.
- It can be taken alone or with a meal.

WHEATGRASS

- Comes from sprouted wheat grain.
- It is a natural detoxifier and helps to speed the release of toxins from the bloodstream.
- Helps to hydrate and energize the cells.
- Helps to maintain balanced pH levels and alkalinize the body.
- Contains powerful enzymes and antioxidants, and helps with digestion.

Using Wheatgrass

- Add 1-3 tsp. of wheatgrass powder to water, juice, or smoothie.
- Can be purchased fresh, which must be juiced.
- Many health markets and fresh squeezed juice bars offer wheatgrass juice.

GOJI BERRIES

- Goji berries have been used in traditional Chinese medicine for thousands of years.
- They are low in calories, fat-free and are loaded with fiber.
- They have a mild tangy taste and are similar in shape and chewy texture to raisins.
- Contain compounds that are naturally anti-inflammatory, anti-fungal, and anti-bacterial.

- Goji berries are packed with vitamin C and beta-carotene.
- Zeaxanthin, a compound found in goji berries, can help protect the retina and improve vision.
- They are known to protect the liver and boost immune function.
- They are rich in antioxidants.

Using Goji Berries

- They can be eaten right out of the bag, added to oatmeal or cereal, included in a trail mix, brewed into tea, or consumed as a juice.

Contraindications: If you are taking blood thinners or medication for diabetes or high blood pressure, talk to your doctor before incorporating goji berries into your diet.

FISH OIL

- Fish oil comes from fish that are rich in omega-3 fatty acid, such as tuna, salmon, sardines, trout and mackerel.
- Consuming fish is a great way to increase your omega-3 intake, however supplementing with fish oil enables you to meet your daily needs without having to chow down on fish everyday.
- Fish oil is highly beneficial for preventing heart disease. It can help to lower blood pressure and triglyceride levels.
- It is a great brain food, as it helps with depression, ADHD, and anxiety.
- Fish oil helps to promote healthy hair, skin and nails.
- Helps reduce inflammation, as well as pain and swelling.
- Promotes optimal fat metabolism and can contribute to weight loss.

Using Fish Oil

- Take 1 tsp. of fish oil daily (at least 1000mg omega-3). *See page 221 for recommended brand.*

ALOE VERA JUICE OR GEL

- Aloe vera is a plant member of the lily family.
- Aloe vera juice is used to promote nutrient absorption, digestive health, immune support and improved overall health.
- It is incredible soothing to the digestive system and helps to reduce symptoms of acid reflux.
- It is anti-inflammatory, anti-bacterial and anti-viral.
- It encourages the release of pepsin, which is a digestive enzyme needed for proper digestion.
- Aloe has natural laxative properties and can help with constipation.
- Helps to detoxify the body.
- It is incredibly healing and moisturizing for the skin - benefits can be seen by taking aloe juice internally or by using it topically on your skin.

What is the Difference Between Aloe Vera Juice and Aloe Vera Gel?

In terms of nutritional value, there is no difference. When used on the skin, the gel can feel a bit more soothing due to its thicker consistency.

Can I Consume that Green Aloe Vera Gel that is Marketed for Sunburns?

No. That stuff contains way too many harsh and unhealthy ingredients, and should never be consumed (or used on your skin for that matter). Look for an aloe vera juice that contains only the aloe plant itself (sometimes citric acid and potassium sorbate will be added as a stabilizer and mold inhibitor – this is okay). It is also important to choose one that is organic.

Contraindications: Consult your doctor before consuming aloe vera if you are pregnant.

Using Aloe Vera

- Drink 2-4 tablespoons as needed (up to eight ounces per day).
- Start slowly if you have never taken aloe before.
- For optimal results, take thirty minutes before each meal.
- Safe for kids, but should be given in a lower dose.
- Store aloe vera juice and/or gel in the fridge after opening for optimal freshness.

* See page 93 for aloe vera lemonade recipe.

COCONUT

It can be confusing trying to understand why we are told to avoid saturated fat, yet are told to consume coconut (which is high in saturated fat), as part of a healthy diet. So, what's the deal? Is coconut good for us or not?

Coconut is in fact a nutritious superfood that is rich in fiber, vitamins and minerals. Research shows that coconut helps to improve insulin secretion and utilization of blood glucose. It helps to slow down rises in blood sugar and helps to reduce sugar cravings. Coconut also helps to provide the body with a quick source of energy and helps to relieve symptoms of chronic fatigue. Coconut is antibacterial and antifungal, and helps to promote a healthy immune system.

There is Such A Thing As Healthy Saturated Fat!

It's true. Coconut has a high saturated fat content. However, the type of saturated fat that it contains is different than the unhealthy kind. What makes the saturated fat in coconut different from other saturated fats is the length of the fatty acid chain it contains.

Research shows that long chain fatty acids are the bad types of saturated fat. This type of fat is found in foods that come from animals, and contributes to high cholesterol and heart disease. Coconut, on the other hand, contains medium chain fatty acids, and comes from a vegetarian source as opposed to an animal. When we consume food containing long chain fatty acids, our bodies store this as fat. This contributes to weight gain, high cholesterol, and can even lead to heart disease and diabetes. On the other hand, when we consume foods with medium chain fatty acids, such as coconut, our bodies do not store it as fat, but rather use it for energy. Instead of promoting weight gain, medium chain fatty acids actually help to promote weight loss and help to lower cholesterol levels.

Using Coconut

- Purchase fresh, whole coconut and consume the meat inside on its own as a snack, include it in smoothies, trail mixes, on top of oatmeal, or in dessert recipes.
- Can also purchase dried, unsweetened coconut to be used the same way as fresh coconut.
- Grated fresh coconut should be stored in the refrigerator, in an airtight container, for up to four days, or frozen for up to six months.
- *Tips for using coconut oil – page 69*
- *Tips for using coconut water – page 114*
- *Tips for using coconut milk – page 62*

SUMMARY

- Include at least one superfood into your daily diet. Do not stick to the same superfoods each day – choose a variety.
- Superfoods contain vitamins, minerals and other nutrients that help to prevent disease and promote overall health and vitality.
- Superfoods include: chia seeds, flax seeds, hemp seeds, cacao, spirulina, wheatgrass, goji berries, fish oil, aloe vera, and coconut.

GUNK-FREE HABIT #14
Get That Body Moving

> **HABIT #14 HOW-TO**: Get at least twenty to thirty minutes of physical exercise each day. Run, walk, skip, swim, lift weights, or even dance in your room. Whatever it is, just keep your body moving!

"If it's important to you, you will find a way. If not, you will find an excuse." - unknown

GET UP AND GET MOVING

If exercise is already a part of your routine, you're one step ahead. If not, it is incredibly important to incorporate some form of physical activity into your daily routine in order to detoxify your system and promote overall better health. Whether you choose to slip on your spandex shorts and head for the gym, follow along to a workout video in your basement, or take a jog around the block, just find a way to get moving.

Daily exercise can help to prevent heart disease, lower blood pressure, lower cholesterol, and help to prevent diabetes, osteoporosis and even cancer. In addition, exercise is a great way to de-stress and re-focus your mind.

The idea is to work hard enough to break a sweat. This will allow your body to detoxify and rid itself of harmful toxins and excess weight.

If you have a membership at a gym or other exercise facility, great! Get on the treadmill, elliptical or bike, attend a class, or do some resistance/weight bearing exercises. If you are not a member and do not have any exercise equipment at home, there is still plenty for you to do. You aren't going to get out of this one so easily - no excuses! There are plenty of highly effective exercises that you can do right in the comfort of your own home.

HOW TO EXERCISE AT HOME

If you do not have access to a treadmill, exercise bike, elliptical or other cardio machine, try some of these exercises:

Jumping Jacks- The traditional exercise of jumping jacks can still be quite challenging. Make sure your core is tight and movements are quick and controlled. Do 3-4 sets of 20-30 jumping jacks.

Step Exercises- Using the stairs, you can do step-ups. Do a few sets of simply stepping up and down one or two stairs. Stepping up onto a coffee table also works, and is a bit tougher (as long as the coffee table is sturdy enough). You can also run up and down the entire flight of stairs for an even more challenging workout.

Squats and lunges- These exercises are not only good for your heart, but are also great for your legs and buttocks. If you want to increase the difficulty of either squats or lunges, hold light weights in your hands while completing the exercise. This will also help to keep you balanced.

Crunches- Crunches are great for building up and strengthening the abdominal muscles. Try challenging yourself by lifting your legs in the air, bicycling your legs, or crossing one leg over the opposite knee, and rotating after each set of five crunches.

Walking- If the weather is nice, take advantage of walking outside. Try walking around your neighborhood at a brisk pace for about twenty to thirty minutes. If you can, challenge yourself to jog, or increase the length of your walk.

Workout Videos- Try following a workout video that guides you through a series of cardio and strength exercises. These can be done in the privacy of your own home and are a great way to stay motivated while exercising.

Dance like Nobody is Watching- Put on your favorite music and have yourself a dance party. Whether it's by yourself or with your family/friends, dancing is a great way to burn some calories, break a sweat, and detoxify the body.

STAY HYDRATED

Avoid reaching for colorful, sugar-filled sports drinks before or after a workout. Many of them contain artificial ingredients, and in fact, actually dehydrate the body even more, due to their high sugar content. Instead of choosing these types of drinks, try some coconut water.

Coconut Water – An All-Natural Sports Drink

- Coconut water is taken from young coconuts that haven't had time to develop coconut milk (which is a mixture of the meat and the water).
- It contains electrolytes, which are mineral ions that your body needs for the regulation of many of its functions, including muscle function, water regulation and nerve transmission.
- The molecular structure of coconut water is identical to human blood plasma, and was even used in World War II to give emergency transfusions to wounded soldiers.
- It is an excellent source of potassium - 600mg of potassium per serving.
  - » Helps with fluid retention, regulates blood pressure and helps to alkalinize the body.
- It does not contain artificial coloring and high fructose corn syrup like many of the sports drinks on the market.
- Coconut water contains less sodium than sports drinks.
- Contains natural sugars, whereas sports drinks contain either refined or artificial sweeteners.
- It's refreshing and delicious!

Choosing a coconut water

Look for a brand of coconut water made without added sugar, and make sure that it is not from concentrate. Choose one that lists pure coconut water as its only ingredient (ascorbic acid may be added – this is okay). If coconut water is flavored, make sure it is flavored with fresh fruit puree, and again, no added sugar.

SUMMARY

- Get at least twenty to thirty minutes of physical exercise each day.
- You do not have to belong to a gym in order to be active. Walk or run outside, walk up and down your stairs, do jumping jacks, crunches, lunges or workout videos at home.
- Re-hydrate after a workout with coconut water instead of artificially made sports drinks. Coconut water is packed with electrolytes, and is naturally sweet without refined or artificial ingredients.

GUNK-FREE HABIT #15
Sip on a Smoothie

> **HABIT #15 HOW-TO:** Consume a healthy smoothie daily, as a snack or as part of a healthy breakfast.

You know that coffee commercial, where strands of steam from the coffee cup penetrate right up the woman's nose, reminding her that the only reason she woke up that morning was to dramatically rip open the dazzling white drapes and sit down with her "I will die if I don't drink you right now", cup of instant coffee?

Well, your morning can look just like that. Except with no steam, no dramatic drape opening and no peaceful music playing in the background (although, the last two are really up to you). You are going to feel just as amazingly energized as the woman in that scene, and the only difference is that your energy will be long lasting, and will not result in a coffee-induced energy crash. Your energy will come from the most amazing, high protein, antioxidant-rich, anti-inflammatory, superfood filled smoothie. Yes, you're right, absolutely nothing like the commercial.

WHY A SMOOTHIE?

One of the best ways to pack a large amount of nutrients into your diet is by making a smoothie. Drinking smoothies enables you to obtain the nutrients from the foods it contains in the most easily absorbed way. After all, we are only as healthy as what our bodies are actually able to absorb. Food in liquid form is much easier for our bodies to digest and absorb, making the potency of the delicious ingredients that much more powerful.

A healthy smoothie should contain vitamins, minerals, protein, fiber and healthy fat. This provides all of the essential ingredients that we need for good health. It provides us with long-lasting energy and helps to keep us feeling full and satisfied throughout the day.

Another great benefit of smoothies is their simplicity. They are simple to make, and take only a few minutes to prepare. They can be taken on-the-go, and are great for those with a busy lifestyle. They can be consumed daily as part of a healthy breakfast, or as an afternoon pick-me-up. They are also great for before or after a workout.

BUILDING YOUR SMOOTHIE

Note: You will require a blender to make your smoothies.

A healthy smoothie should include a source of protein (from protein powder, yogurt or kefir and/or protein-rich superfoods), a source of fiber (from fruits, vegetables, whole grains or superfoods), and a source of healthy fat.

A smoothie should include ingredients from each of the following categories:

Liquid (1 cup) – choose one or combine them to equal one cup

- Water or coconut water.
- Milk alternative (hemp milk, rice milk, almond milk, coconut milk).
- Fresh squeezed juices (lemon, orange, apple, pomegranate, etc.).

Thickener

Depending on how you like your smoothie, you may want to include a thickening agent to make it thick and creamy. If you prefer a lighter smoothie, you do not have to add a thickener. However, many of the thickening agents are packed with beneficial nutrients and help to increase the nutrient density of your smoothies. Thickeners include:

- Plain, unsweetened Greek yogurt or kefir (1/2 cup)
- Ice (1/2 cup)
- Avocado (¼ - ½)
- Banana (½ - 1 full banana)
- Natural nut or seed butter (1-2 tbsp.)

Fruits and Vegetables

The beauty of smoothies is that you can pack a whole bunch of fruits and vegetables into your diet in one glass. The great thing about adding leafy greens (kale, spinach, etc.) into your smoothies is that you don't even taste them, but are able to reap all of their nutritional benefits.

You can use fresh or frozen fruit in your smoothies, and all fruits and vegetables are fair game! Some suggested fruits and vegetables include:

- Blueberries
- Raspberries
- Strawberries
- Pineapple
- Papaya
- Apple
- Pear
- Grapes
- Pomegranate
- Dates
- Banana
- Kiwi fruit
- Mango
- Kale
- Spinach
- Parsley
- Swiss chard
- Cucumber
- Pumpkin
- Sweet potato

Protein Powder - Optional

It is important to get enough protein in your diet, and healthy smoothies are a great way to meet your daily protein needs. Not all smoothies need to include protein powder, however, it is a great option if you are consuming a smoothie as a meal replacement or before/after a workout.

When choosing a protein powder, always look for one that is free of refined sugar, artificial flavors and artificial colors *(see page 78 for more on protein powders)*.

Superfoods and Natural Sweeteners

Sweeteners (amount is based on desired taste)

- Pure maple syrup
- Raw honey
- Bee pollen
- Stevia
- Dates
- Coconut sugar

Superfoods

- Chia seeds
- Flax seeds
- Hemp seeds
- Flax seed, hemp seed or chia seed oils
- Fish oil
- Spirulina powder
- Cacao
- Matcha powder
- Maca
- Bee pollen
- Raw honey
- Fresh coconut
- Dried coconut
- Raw nuts (almonds, hazelnuts, pecans, Brazil nuts, etc...)
- Wheatgrass
- Aloe vera juice or gel

KEEP YOUR SMOOTHIE HEALTHY

It is important to make healthy smoothies that are nourishing to the body and help to promote good health. It is best to **avoid** refined sugar, artificial sweeteners, and other artificial ingredients when making your smoothies.

Have fun with your smoothies and play around to see what works and what doesn't. Experiment with flavours and ingredients.

SUMMARY:

- Consume a healthy smoothie daily as a snack or as part of a healthy breakfast.
- A healthy smoothie should contain foods rich in vitamins, minerals, protein, fiber, and healthy fat.
- Smoothies provide long-lasting energy.
- To build your own smoothie recipe, include a liquid, a thickening agent, fruits and vegetables, a source of protein, superfoods and natural sweeteners.
- Avoid refined sugar, artificial sweeteners and other artificial ingredients when making your smoothie.

GUNK-FREE HABIT #16
Make Friends with Probiotics

> **HABIT #16 HOW-TO:** Consume probiotic-rich foods and/or supplement with a high quality probiotic supplement daily, in order to maintain a healthy gut.

MEET YOUR NEW FRIENDS

It's time to invite some "friendly" bacteria to the party! That's right, our good friends, probiotics.

Probiotics, also referred to as "friendly" or "good" bacteria, are live microorganisms that are found in the human digestive tract. They are known to help restore the proper balance of good and bad bacteria in the intestines, promote healthy immune function, strengthen the digestive tract, aid in the digestion and absorption of food, help with elimination and prevent constipation, reduce allergy symptoms and contribute to overall well being.

Often, we do not have enough of these good bacteria present in our digestive systems naturally. The use of antibiotics, consumption of processed and refined foods, coffee consumption, and stress, all deplete our natural "friendly" bacteria. Probiotic supplements and/or probiotic rich foods are recommended in order to restore proper levels.

PROBIOTIC-RICH FOODS

Consuming probiotic-rich foods is a great way to increase the levels of "friendly" bacteria in your gut. Fermented foods such as **yogurt, kefir, miso, tempeh, kombucha, and sauerkraut** are excellent sources of probiotics.

Kefir

Kefir is a fermented drink made with cow, goat, or sheep milk and kefir grains. It is a probiotic-rich, creamy product, similar to yogurt. The difference between kefir and yogurt is that kefir contains beneficial yeast as well as the friendly bacteria found in yogurt. The yeasts used to make kefir (Saccharomyces kefir and Torula kefir) ferment the lactose, which makes it easy to digest, and in some cases, even for those suffering from lactose intolerance.

Tempeh

Tempeh is made from fermented soybeans. Although heavily processed and genetically modified soy is not good for us, tempeh actually offers many health benefits, due to the fact that it is fermented. Tempeh is a great source of protein, and is perfect for vegetarians, vegans and omnivores. Animal protein is high in saturated fat and cholesterol, whereas tempeh does not contain any cholesterol and is much lower in fat. In fact, the soy protein found in tempeh has been shown to help lower cholesterol levels.

Tempeh is not only a good source of protein, but also a great source of dietary fiber. It contains healthy probiotics that help to promote proper bowel function and reduce symptoms of gas, bloating, diarrhea and constipation.

Using Tempeh

- Tempeh is sold in the freezer section of the grocery store. It is commonly sold in health food stores or local markets.
- Tempeh must be defrosted before being consumed. Defrost in the refrigerator or place in a bowl of cold water.
- Refrigerated tempeh can be kept in the refrigerator for up to ten days.
- You may notice a white layer covering the tempeh and black or gray spots. This is completely normal and is part of the fermentation process.
- Tempeh is rather flavorless on its own, however, it absorbs the flavours of the foods in which it is cooked or marinated.
- It can be eaten hot or cold and served with vegetables, rice, quinoa, salads, in sauces, in sandwiches, in chili, or any way you like.

Delicious tempeh recipe on page 188.

Miso

Miso, meaning, "fermented beans", comes from fermented soybeans. It is generally found as a thick paste, and the color and taste vary depending on the fermentation process.

Miso contains antioxidants like zinc, manganese, and phenolic acid. It is also rich in tryptophan (precursor for the feel good hormone, serotonin), vitamin k (helps with bone formation), phosphorus, copper, and omega-3 fatty acids.

Miso contains lactic acid bacteria and lactobacillus, known as "friendly bacteria", which support our intestinal micro flora. Therefore, the consumption of miso helps to protect against diseases of the digestive tract. It is also rich in fiber and protein.

Using Miso

- Store miso in the refrigerator in a tightly sealed container. It can keep in the fridge for up to one year.
- Darker miso has a stronger flavour, while light colored miso has a more mild taste and is more delicate.
- Miso can be used in soups, dressings, light sauces, stir-fry, sandwiches, marinades, and dips.
- **Miso soup** – simply heat miso paste and water over low heat. Add in toppings such as mushrooms, onions, carrots and radishes.
- Make sure to buy certified organic miso, as soybeans are highly genetically modified when they are not organic. Check the label to ensure there are no additives, such a MSG.

Sauerkraut

Sauerkraut is fermented cabbage made by lactic fermentation. Cabbage naturally contains the necessary bacteria and yeast required for the fermentation process and only requires the addition of salt to kick-start the process.

The fermentation process produces substances called isothiocyanates, which may help prevent tumors and are anti-cancerous. Unpasteurized sauerkraut is full of lactobacillus bacteria, which is beneficial for gut health, immune health and digestion.

Saurkraut is rich in enzymes which help to break down the food we eat and speed up metabolic processes. It is rich in fiber, and has been known to relieve upset stomachs and constipation.

Using Sauerkraut

- Choose unpasteurized or raw cultured sauerkraut. This means that the sauerkraut has never been heated. Heating destroys the naturally occurring digestive enzymes and "good" bacteria.
- Choose one made without vinegar or preservatives.
- Choose an organic variety when possible.
- Sauerkraut is commonly eaten alongside meat dishes, and can be added to sandwiches, salads, or eaten straight out of the jar.

PROBIOTIC SUPPLEMENTS

Supplementing with a high quality probiotic daily is recommended. It is important to ensure that the supplement you choose contains enough friendly bacteria to do your body any good. Choosing a brand with over ten billion live organisms is beneficial. You should also ensure that the brand you choose is from the refrigerator section at your local health food store. Probiotics are made up of live organisms, and therefore must be kept cool in order to survive.

Make sure to follow the instructions on the bottle. Take 2-3 times per day with a meal, and store in the fridge. Take for thirty days (or longer for maintenance).

SUMMARY:

- Consume probiotic-rich foods and/or supplement with a high-quality probiotic supplement daily, in order to maintain a healthy gut.
- Probiotic-rich foods include, kefir, yogurt, miso, tempeh, kombucha and sauerkraut.
- When supplementing with probiotics, make sure to choose one with over ten billion live organisms and one that is stored in the refrigerator section of your local health food store.

GUNK-FREE HABIT #17
Spice Up Your Life

> **HABIT #17 HOW-TO**: Add some herbs and spices to your food for a more fragrant, nutrient-rich meal.

Herbs and spices don't only make our food taste delicious, but they also provide amazingly powerful health benefits. Adding a variety of herbs and spices to your food helps to keep your palate happy, while helping to promote better health. No herb or spice is off limits, so play around with different kinds to see which ones you like the most. The same bowl of quinoa can taste quite different when topped with cinnamon than it does when cooked with garlic. Herbs and spices help to change up the flavor of your food, so that you don't get bored of eating the same thing too often.

Try to incorporate all (or at least some) of the herbs and spices listed below into your daily diet. These particular items have extremely powerful healing benefits and are quite versatile in terms of their uses.

CINNAMON

- Cinnamon is a delicious spice that comes from the inner bark of the tropical cinnamon tree.
- It is powerful in helping to lower blood sugar and is incredibly beneficial for diabetics.
- Adding cinnamon to a carbohydrate-rich food can help to decrease its impact on your blood sugar levels.
- By helping to balance blood sugar, cinnamon actually helps to promote weight loss.
- Cinnamon helps to boost immune function.

Using Cinnamon

- Consume ½ - 1 tsp. daily.
- Add to oatmeal, yogurt, tea, desserts, sweet potatoes, and toast.
- Can be purchased in sticks or powder.

TURMERIC

- Turmeric comes from the root of the Curcuma longa plant.
- It is often used in powder form.
- Turmeric is bight yellow in color.
- It has a warm, bitter taste.
- It is rich in iron and manganese.
- Turmeric root is often used to treat arthritis, diarrhea, bloating, fever, and headaches.
- It is a natural painkiller.
- Has antibacterial properties and is a natural liver detoxifier.
- Has been shown to stop the growth of new blood vessels in tumors.
- Research shows that the active ingredient, curcumin, helps to provide a well-tolerated, and effective treatment for inflammatory bowel disease (IBD) such as Crohn's and ulcerative colitis.
- Helps to reduce inflammation – has been shown to be as effective as anti-inflammatory medications.

Using Turmeric

- Turmeric can be added to brown rice, steamed vegetables, curry, dips, lentils, and salad dressing, among other dishes.
- Turmeric powder should kept in a cool, dark and dry place

Contraindications: Turmeric should not be used by anyone with gallstones or bile obstruction. If you are pregnant, consult your doctor before using turmeric. Turmeric can slow blood clotting and therefore should not be used at least two weeks before a scheduled surgery.

GARLIC

- Garlic is a member of the Allium genus and classified as Allium sativa.
- Fresh garlic helps to lower total cholesterol, while raising HDL (good cholesterol) and lowering LDL (bad cholesterol).
- Has anti-inflammatory properties.

- Helps to boost immune function and protect against viruses and bacteria.
- Garlic contains the enzyme allicin, which is an antioxidant that helps to protect against cancer and heart disease.

Using Garlic

- Garlic is available fresh or in powder form.
- When choosing fresh garlic, select one that looks plump, dry and firm.
- Do not store garlic in the fridge. Keep it in a cool, dark place.
- Add 1-2 cloves of garlic to salad dressing, stir fry, soup, meat, poultry or fish.
- Fresh, raw garlic contains the highest level of nutrients and carries the most benefit.
- Do not cook garlic for too long or at too high a temperature. It can become fairly bitter and loses many of its vital nutrients.

> **Gunk-Free Tip**: To help reduce high cholesterol, consume one clove of fresh garlic everyday.

Garlic Stink No More!

Garlic can leave your hands smelling for days. To eliminate this odor, rinse your hands with a mixture of salt and lemon juice, and then wash your hands with soap and water.

GINGER

- Ginger is the underground rhizome of the ginger plant.
- It helps to alleviate inflammation in the digestive system and thus helps to promote better digestion.
- It is a powerful herb for detoxification.
- Ginger contains volatile oils that help to reduce symptoms of motion sickness such as dizziness, vomiting, cold sweats and nausea.
- Great for reducing bloating and gas.

Purchasing Ginger

- Ginger can be purchased fresh or in powder form.
- Fresh ginger has a stronger flavor and is more nutrient dense.
- Purchase ginger that is firm and smooth.

Using Ginger

- Ginger can be grated or chopped.
- Ginger can be added to tea or hot water with some lemon, salad dressing, marinades, grilled vegetables and stir-fry.
- Ginger has a pungent, spicy taste.
- Unpeeled ginger can be stored in the fridge or freezer.

PARSLEY

- Parsley is a diuretic and therefore helps to flush out the body and aid with weight loss.
- It is a powerful digestive aid and helps to promote elimination.
- It has antioxidant and antibacterial properties and helps to lower cholesterol and increase calcium levels in the body.
- Parsley helps to cleanse the palate and is often consumed after a meal as a breath freshener.
- Parsley is rich in vitamin K, which is necessary for the synthesis of osteocalcin, a protein that strengthens the composition of our bones.
- Parsley is packed with antioxidants that help to protect the body against free radical damage.
- It has anti-inflammatory qualities.
- It helps to bind heavy metals and flush them out of the body.
- It is rich in vitamins C and vitamin A.

Using Parsley

- Parsley can be added to salad, quinoa or rice, soups, sauces, on top of fish or chicken, or eaten on its own.
- Fresh parsley can be stored in the fridge for up to two weeks or can be frozen for up to six months.

WARM UP AND SOOTHE WITH PARSLEY AND GINGER TEA

Gunk-Free Tip: Drink ¼ cup of homemade parsley and ginger tea each morning (or at a time that is convenient for you).

Parsley and ginger tea helps to cleanse and detoxify the body in a powerful way. It helps to flush out the kidneys and improve their function, aid with weight loss, as well as reduce gas and bloating.

This simple practice can have tremendous results, so try to include it into your daily routine a few times per week.

How to Make Parsley and Ginger Tea

- Purchase fresh parsley (organic) from the store.
- Rinse parsley, and boil in 1 quart of water for 3 minutes. Strain out the liquid into a mug, add fresh ground ginger and drink ¼ cup.
- Discard of the parsley in the compost.
- The remaining liquid can be refrigerated for 3-4 days.

Note: This can be quite powerful. If you notice any signs of digestive upset, reduce the amount of ginger, and slowly increase as the days go on.

SUMMARY:

- Add some herbs and spices to your food for a more fragrant, nutrient-rich meal.
- Incorporate cinnamon, garlic, ginger, turmeric, and parsley into your daily diet. These spices contain amazing healing properties.
- Drink ¼ cup of homemade parsley and ginger tea daily when possible.

GUNK-FREE HABIT #18
Brush Your Skin, Dry

You brush your teeth and (likely) brush your hair, but have you ever tried brushing your skin? Daily dry skin brushing enables you to rid your skin and body of impurities. You're going to love this!

Dry skin brushing enables you to de-gunk your body from the outside in. The skin is the largest, most important eliminative organ in the body and is responsible for one quarter of the body's detoxification each day. The dry brushing technique deals with detoxification of the skin and is a great way to stimulate your organs as it provides a gentle internal massage.

BENEFITS OF DRY SKIN BRUSHING

- Removes cellulite
- Cleanses the lymphatic system
- Removes dead skin layers
- Strengthens the immune system
- Tightens the skin preventing premature aging
- Tones the muscles
- Stimulates circulation
- Improves the function of the nervous system
- Helps digestion

WHAT YOU NEED

To dry brush, use a soft natural fiber brush with a long handle so that you are able to reach all areas of your body. A loofah, sponge, or a rough towel can also be used. Most nylon and synthetic fiber brushes are too sharp and may damage skin.

TIPS AND TRICKS

- Always dry brush your body before you shower or bathe. Showering after a good skin brushing will help to wash off the dead skin.
- You can do the brushing head-to-toe or toe-to-head, the order you choose does not matter.
- When brushing the legs, start from the bottom of your feet and brush upwards.
- When brushing the arms, start from the hands towards the shoulders.
- When brushing the torso, brush in an upward direction.
- Brush the skin in a circular motion, always towards the heart - this helps drain the lymph back to your heart.
- Once you have brushed your skin and showered, dry off and massage your skin with pure plant oils such as olive, avocado, apricot, almond, sesame, coconut, or cocoa butter.

Important: Stroking away from your heart puts extra pressure on the valves within the veins and lymph vessels and can cause ruptured vessels and varicose veins. Always brush towards the heart.

GUNK-FREE HABIT #19
Undress Your Stress

UGHHHHHH!

We are all stressed, that's simply a part of life. We have jobs, families, and perhaps even children to look after. We have lists of things to accomplish, places to be, and things to do. But, despite all of that, it is essential to take some time each day for YOU!

You will never be completely free of stress, however, by implementing some stress-busting techniques, you will have the ability to cope with your stress much better.

Before learning how to cope with stress, it is important to first understand how stress actually affects your body and your overall health.

HOW DOES STRESS AFFECT OUR HEALTH?

Stress can trigger what is known as the fight-or-flight response (the body's response to perceived threat or danger). During this reaction, certain hormones called adrenalin and cortisol are released. When released, they work to speed the heart rate, slow digestion, shunt blood flow, and provide your body with a burst of energy and strength.

Originally, this fight or flight response was named for its ability to enable us to physically fight or run away when faced with danger. Now, however, it is activated in situations where neither response is appropriate, like in traffic, line-ups, or during a stressful day at work.

When the perceived "threat" is gone, the relaxation response is designed to enable our bodies to return to normal function – a calm state of being. In times of chronic stress, when your body does not have the opportunity to slow down, the relaxation response is not activated, causing damage to the body.

Too much stress over time weakens the adrenal glands and causes them to release these fight or flight hormones without warning. This leads to lack of energy, fatigue, various aches and pains, headaches, emotional disorders such as anxiety, depression, and sleep disturbances, ulcers, lower abdominal cramps, irritable bowel syndrome, heart conditions, and high blood pressure.

In order to manage stress, it is important to follow a healthy diet, get regular exercise, incorporate some stress busting techniques into your daily routine, as well as make time for uninterrupted relaxation.

KICK STRESS IN THE BUTT!

Sleep

Proper sleep is essential in order to restore our bodies and refresh our minds. When we are too stressed, we cannot sleep. When we are not sleeping, our bodies do not have time to recover and rejuvenate so we are unable to effectively cope and recover from our stress. This is a vicious cycle.

When we sleep, immune enhancing chemicals are released which help to protect our immune systems and improve overall health. Without adequate sleep, our natural killer cells (cells which destroy germs) do not function optimally.

It is important to get between six to eight hours of sleep per night. This allows your body to go through the proper sleep cycles and leads to feeling energized and focused in the morning. The quality of sleep had is just as important as the amount of time slept. Sleeping from one o'clock a.m. to nine o'clock a.m. is not thought to be as restorative as sleeping from ten o'clock p.m. to six o'clock a.m. The key is to get to bed by ten o'clock p.m. for the most peaceful, restorative sleep.

Gunk-Free Tips for Getting Better Sleep:

- **Sleep in complete darkness** - Even the smallest amount of light can lead to difficulty falling asleep and poor overall sleep. Turn off all lights (indoor and outdoor), televisions, and computers in your bedroom.
- **Keep cool** – Better sleep is achieved in a cooler environment. Turn your thermostat down at bedtime and avoid wearing anything that makes you feel too hot.
- **Set a kitchen curfew** – Eating close to bedtime can result in poor sleep and may even result in excessive trips to the bathroom throughout the night. Avoid eating at least two hours before bed to avoid indigestion and restlessness while you sleep.
- **Clear your mind** – Often, our thoughts can prevent us from falling asleep easily and may even keep us up throughout the night. Practice deep breathing or meditation before bed to help calm the mind and body. Write down your thoughts before bed and get back to them in the morning. Good sleep provides clarity and focus for the day ahead.
- **Have sex** – Having sex (with a partner or even by yourself) releases feel good hormones, which help to calm the nervous system and promote relaxation.

Magnesium

Magnesium is a mineral required for more than three hundred biochemical reactions inside the body. It is also needed to protect and support our nervous system, and enables us to relax and handle stress much better. In fact, magnesium is known as the anti-stress mineral. Our bodies don't produce it, so it is essential to get adequate magnesium through whole foods and even supplementation in some cases.

A magnesium deficiency can contribute to insomnia, bone and joint pain, muscle spasms, anxiety and panic attacks, headaches and heart arrhythmias. It is important to consume a magnesium-rich diet and even supplement with magnesium in order to ensure that you are meeting your daily needs.

Magnesium Rich Foods

Include some of these magnesium rich foods in your diet:

- Bananas
- Almonds
- Figs
- Beans
- Oat bran
- Pumpkin seeds
- Brown rice
- Spinach

Supplementing with Magnesium

Adults should be getting between 400-600mg of magnesium per day.

Magnesium can be taken in pill, liquid or powder form.

Recommended brand: Natural Calm Magnesium Citrate Powder. Follow instructions on bottle.

Contraindications: Consult your doctor before supplementing with magnesium if you have kidney disease or taking heart medication.

B Vitamins

There are eight essential B vitamins that our bodies need. These vitamins are necessary for immune and nervous system function, energy production, normal growth and development, mental health and stress.

A B-complex vitamin is comprised of eight essential B vitamins and several related substances. The eight vitamins are vitamin B1 (thiamine), vitamin B2 (riboflavin), vitamin B3 (niacin), vitamin B5 (pantothenic acid), vitamin B6 (pyridoxine), vitamin B7 (biotin), vitamin B9 (folic acid), and vitamin B12 (cyanocobalamin).

B5 is often referred to as the "anti-stress vitamin". It is critical to the manufacturing of stress-related hormones produced in the adrenal glands.

B6 helps to produce the "feel good" chemical called serotonin. Changes in serotonin levels can alter mood and affect a person's ability to cope with stress.

B1, B2, B3 are helpful in dealing with physical stress.

If supplementing with B vitamins, choose a high quality B-complex vitamin, made without added fillers and chemicals. **Take a 50 mg complex one to two times daily.** Visit your local health food store to find a brand that works for you.

There are also a number of food sources that contain these essential B vitamins.

Try incorporating some of these vitamin B rich foods into your diet:

- Beans
- Liver
- Wheat bran
- Bananas
- Oats
- Turkey
- Avocados
- Salmon
- Lentils
- Spinach
- Turnip greens
- Eggs
- Whole-grains

Yoga

Yoga has a calming effect on the nervous system, and in particular, the brain. It helps to increase blood circulation to the sleep center in the brain, which has the effect of normalizing the sleep cycle. Yoga also increases the elimination of toxins from the body and rejuvenates the entire body.

Attending a yoga class at your local yoga studio is a great way to de-stress, however, yoga can also be done right in the comfort of your own home. It allows you to take some time each day to check in with yourself, breathe and sweat out unwanted toxins.

Smell Your Way to Calmness

Aromatherapy is great for calming the mind, improving mood, increasing alertness and focus, and providing a sense of overall health and well-being. Aromatherapy is based on using volatile plant materials, known as essential oils, to help relieve tension and stress.

Essential oils can be used in a number of different ways. When choosing essential oils, it is important to purchase food grade oils, as these can be taken internally and are safest to use. These oils can be added to herbal teas, used in a bath, or applied directly to the skin. When using essential oils on the skin, add a few drops of your favorite scent to a carrier oil (avocado oil, coconut oil, shea butter or other oil/unscented lotion of choice), and massage into the skin. You can also place a few drops of the essential oil onto your palm or behind your ear.

Diffusing essential oils in the home, office, or car is also beneficial. There are a number of different diffusers on the market, so choose one that suits you best.

Try some of the following essential oils:

- **Chamomile** – Effective antispasmodic and nerve sedative. Helps to combat stress.
- **Lavender** – Relaxes and relieves stress.
- **Rosemary** – Stimulates the mind.
- **Sandalwood** – Great for insomnia and depression.
- **Lemon** - Calming, helps relieve mental fatigue, nervousness and nervous tension.
- **Peppermint** – Provides relief from stress, depression and mental exhaustion. It is also effective against anxiety and restlessness.

You Time

You time is one of the most important things you can do for yourself, your health and your stress levels - and it's so super simple to do. All you have to do is schedule at least twenty minutes each day just for YOU. This time is for you to relax and do what you enjoy, away from everyone and everything else that might need, or want, your attention. Read, walk around the block, meditate, take a bath or get a massage. Just do whatever it is that you like to do, without distraction. This time is so incredibly important as it enables you to check in with yourself and unwind. You will find that just twenty minutes a day makes a huge difference.

Just Let It Go

> *"Incredible change happens in your life when you decide to take control of what you do have power over instead of craving control over what you don't"* – Steve Maraboli

Part of living gunk-free is freeing your mind from clutter. Our own thoughts can be our worst enemies, and without even realizing it, can contribute to poor health. When we focus too much on things that are out of our control or simply don't matter in the long run, we take time away from focusing on what does matter – our health and happiness.

The things we can't control are the things that often end up controlling us; they control our thoughts and affect our mood. Holding on to things, holds you back. It holds you back from feeling free and achieving greater things. Holding on to failed relationships, a job that you just don't love, or things that you might have said or done that wish you had said or done differently, all lead to gunky-ness in your mind.

When you let go of things, an entire world of possibilities opens up. When we focus our energy so much on something, it takes away from other things that we could be focusing on – finding new love, getting the job of our dreams, or enjoying the simple things, like time with family and friends.

It's so easy to get caught up in our failures, misfortunes, and daily struggles. It's easy to let our thoughts control us – they are powerful enough to ruin an entire day – a day that you will never get back. It's hard to see the light at the end of the tunnel sometimes, but just know that it does exist. When we let go and trust that things will work themselves out, that gunky feeling simply melts away. We feel lighter, more energized, and free.

How to De-Gunk Your Mind

- **Write things down** – Our minds can become overwhelmed with thoughts and ideas, and can become chaotic. Writing things down and creating lists helps to calm the mind, and enables you to organize your thoughts and ideas in a logical way. Writing things down also helps to prevent the possibility of forgetting your brilliant thoughts.

- **Get it off your chest** – Sometimes we have conversations in our head that are intended for another person. The best way to settle the argument or conversation in your head is to actually have that conversation with the intended person. Once you are able to express your thoughts, the fear of having that conversation fades away. Even if the outcome is not as you had hoped, getting it off your chest brings a sense of lightness and relief.

- **Accept things as they are** – Sometimes you just have to say, "It is what it is". Throw your hands up and accept whatever circumstance comes your way. The great thing about accepting is that it enables you to move on. When you are open to moving on, amazing things happen.

- **Be patient** – Wanting it all is great – it means that you have drive and passion. However, it's also extremely overwhelming and exhausting. There are only so many hours in the day and so much that one person can take on at one time. Focus on one thing at a time and decide what is most important. Everything you want to do in your life can be yours, but only when the time is right and you are ready.

SUMMARY:

- In order to effectively manage stress, it is important to follow a healthy diet, get regular exercise, and make time for uninterrupted relaxation.
- It is important to get between six to eight hours of sleep every night. Getting to sleep by ten o'clock p.m. is beneficial.
- Magnesium is the anti-stress mineral. Consume magnesium rich foods such as bananas, figs, almonds and spinach. Supplement with between 400-600mg of magnesium per day.
- B vitamins are needed for stress management. Vitamin B rich foods include, beans, oats, avocados, salmon, whole grains and lentils.
- Practicing yoga and making time for yourself is a great way to de-stress. Take at least twenty minutes each day for *you*.
- Essential oils such as chamomile, lavender, rosemary and lemon help to calm the nervous system and combat stress.
- Let things go, focus on you, get your thoughts and feeling off your chest and accept things as they are. De-gunking your mind is a vital part of living gunk-free.

GUNK-FREE HABIT #20
De-Gunk Your Beauty Care and Household Cleaners

> **HABIT #20 HOW-TO**: Replace some of your conventional beauty care and household cleaning products with more natural alternatives, or try making some of your own products at home.

Just because our skin is on the outside of our bodies, does not mean that it should be treated any differently than the inside. In fact, what goes on our skin is absorbed through our pores and goes directly into our bodies and bloodstreams. This means, that whatever ingredients are lurking in the lotions, creams and beauty products used on your skin, are in fact being directly absorbed into your body. Now, you would never ingest harsh chemicals, coal tar dyes, parabens, or petroleum, so why use it on your skin? The chemicals found in skin care and other beauty products have been linked to serious health conditions such as cancer, reproductive dysfunction, hormone disruption and genetic mutations. Known carcinogens, pesticides and other industrial chemicals (plasticizers, degreasers and surfactants) are used in cosmetics.

An interesting exercise is to investigate the ingredients in your most-used health and beauty products. Take a peek at the list of ingredients and compare your list to the list below. How many of your products contain these harsh chemicals?

Going completely chemical-free is not for everyone, however, everyone can benefit from at least reducing the amount of chemicals used on a daily basis. Even changing two or three of your most-used products to more natural alternatives will help to make a significant difference.

A GUNK-FILLED CHEMICAL COCKTAIL – WHAT'S REALLY LURKING IN YOUR BEAUTY PRODUCTS AND HOUSEHOLD CLEANERS?

BHA (butylated hydroxyanisole) **and BHT** (butylated hydroxytoluene): These synthetic antioxidants are used in common cosmetic products as preservatives. They can be found in moisturizers, makeup, skin creams and lipstick. BHA and BHT are known to disrupt hormone function, cause allergic reactions, cause skin reactions, and increase the risk of cancer.

Coal Tar Dyes: Coal tar dyes are considered potential cancer causing agents and can contain concentration of heavy metals. These chemicals are derived from petroleum and can be found in hair dyes, soaps, and lipstick, and can have potential toxic effects on the brain.

Dibutyl Phthalate: Phthalates are most commonly used to soften plastics but can be found in a number of cosmetic and household products such as nail polish, hair dye and fragrances. In laboratory experiments, it has been shown to contribte to developmental defects, endocrine imbalances, reduced sperm count and reproductive defects. Reesarch shows that they may cause liver and kidney failure.

Parabens: Parabens are preservatives used in cosmetic products, such as skin creams, shaving creams, shampoo, and conditioner, to prevent the formation of mold. The most common forms include methylparaben, butylparaben and propylparaben. Once they penetrate the skin, they can lead to hormone imbalances and interfere with reproductive function. Parabens absorbed by the skin are not metabolized by the body, but rather travel directly into the blood stream, affecting our organs.

Parfum (fragrance) or Perfum: Parfum is a term used to describe a combination of fragrance ingredients. Over three thousand chemicals can be included to produce fragrance. Products that commonly contain fragrance or parfum include perfume, calogne, deodorant, soap, shampoo, laundry detergant, dish soap, air fresheners, and cleaning products.

Parfum has been linked to a number of negative health effects such as cancer, neurotoxicity, allergies and asthma.

Siloxanes: Look for ingredients ending in "siloxane" or "methicone". These chemicals appear in a variety of cosmetics to soften, smooth and moisten. They are added to hair products for faster drying time, deodorants for easier application, moisturizers and facial treatments. They have been suspected to cause endocrine disruption and reproductive toxicity.

Sodium Laureth Sulfate: Can be referred to as SLES or its relative sodium lauryl sulfate. SLES or SLS are added to products to make them foam and bubble. These include, shampoos, facial cleansers, shower gels, toothhpaste, bubble bath, and dish soap. They have been linked to skin irritation including, eczema and psorisis, as well as the development of cancer.

Ammonia can be found in glass cleaners, and many other household cleaning products.

Sodium Fluoride is found in toothpaste and also rat poisoning. Enough said.

GUNK-FREE, DO-IT-YOURSELF NATURAL BEAUTY CARE

- **Skin moisturizer or hair treatment:** After your shower or bath, apply coconut oil directly to your skin or put it on the ends of your hair or on your scalp.
- **Exfoliate** in the shower or bath with a mixture of sea salt and olive oil.
- **Moisturizer:** Use olive oil, almond oil, avocado oil, walnut oil, or other healthy oil as a moisturizer in the shower.
- **Bath time:** Add 1 cup of Epsom salts to your bath for a soothing and muscle relaxing experience. Can also add a few drops of essential oil (lavender, lemon, peppermint) with 1 cup of olive oil.

BODY LOTION

Peppermint Body Lotion

Ingredients

1/2 cup of coconut oil
2 tablespoons of shaved beeswax
2-3 tablespoons of water
10 drops of peppermint essential oil – or oil of your choice

Instructions

- Place coconut oil into stainless steel bowl.
- Add the shaved beeswax.
- Using a double boiler (sauce pan filled with water with the stainless bowl on top), melt the coconut oil and beeswax over medium/high heat.
- Pour 2-3 tablespoons of room temperature water into your blender (can use a hand blender) and begin blending on high speed with the lid on.
- Slowly pour the oil/beeswax mixture into the water. It will begin to emulsify and form a white lotion.
- Add peppermint essential oil (or oil of your choice – lavender is nice too).
- Can add one capsule or a few drops of vitamin E oil.
- Pour lotion into a glass jar or container for storing.
- Apply daily or as needed.

FACEMASKS

Facemask Instructions

- Choose your preferred facemask recipe.
- Place ingredients in bowl and mix together.
- Apply to face for 15-30 minutes.

- Remove using warm water.
- Pat dry.
- Can apply coconut oil to skin after facemask is used for added hydration.

Yogurt and Honey Face Mask

> Yogurt – 1 tablespoon
> Raw Honey – 1 tablespoon
> Coconut oil – 1 tablespoon

Coconut and Honey Face Mask

> Raw honey – 1 tablespoon
> Coconut oil – 1 tablespoon

Cooling Avocado Face Mask

> Avocado pulp (medium ripe) – ½ of the fruit
> 1 tbsp. aloe vera juice or gel
> 1 egg white – tightens the skin
> Raw honey – 1 tablespoon
> Coconut oil – 1 tablespoon

Oats and Honey Face Mask

> 2 tbsp. cooked oats (either in water or coconut milk)
> 1 tsp. raw honey
> Good for sensitive skin, moisturizing, calms skin and reduces redness

Silky Almond Scrub

> 2 tbsp. plain yogurt
> 2 tbsp. raw or manuka honey
> 1 tbsp. almond meal
> The almond granules will help to exfoliate

HAIR CARE

Apple Cider Vinegar

1 tbsp. apple cider vinegar

Using a spray bottle, spray over hair for added shine. Will also help to remove any hair products used in your hair.

Avocado Hair Treatment

1 tsp. avocado oil or crush a fresh avocado with a drop of olive oil.

Leave mixture in your hair for one hour before rinsing.

Hair Strengthener

1 tbsp. coconut oil

1 egg white

Mix together and apply to damp hair. Let it sit for 30 minutes to one hour before rinsing.

HEALTHY HOME, HEALTHY YOU!

Household cleaning products are filled with harsh chemicals, and as soon as they are sprayed into the air or used to dust the furniture, they are being absorbed into your body. The chemical-filled products used to clean kitchen counters or dishes may be effective in removing bacteria and stuck-on-food, but all at a large cost to our health.

If only making small changes to your home cleaning routine, start with the products used in the kitchen or on any surface where food is prepared and/or eaten. The products used to clean these areas can leach into your food, and in turn end up in your body.

Watch out for ingredients such as ammonia, coal tar dyes, sodium hydroxide, propylene glycol, and other unpronounceable chemical names. These items are often found in household cleaners and can result in irritation to the eyes, skin and lungs.

GUNK-FREE, DO-IT-YOURSELF NATURAL HOUSEHOLD CLEANERS

Natural anti-bacterial cleaning agents: white vinegar, baking soda, borax, lemon, salt and essential oils.

Toilet bowl, shower, sink and oven cleaner: Sprinkle baking soda onto the area to be cleaned. Soak a sponge in vinegar and scrub area to remove build-up and grime.

Floor cleaner: Scrub **tile floors** with a mixture of one part water and one part white vinegar. For **other floor surfaces**, use eight times the amount of water as vinegar and add a few drops of fresh lemon or essential oil.

Kitchen counters: Use a mixture of one part vinegar to three parts water. Add a few drops of fresh lemon.

All-purpose and glass cleaner: Mix 1 cup white vinegar with 8 cups water. Can add a few drops of lemon or essential oil for a nice smell. Can also add baking soda for tougher spots.

Drain cleaner: Use a mixture of 1 cup baking soda and 1 cup vinegar. Pour down the drain and wait fifteen to twenty minutes. Then, pour boiling water down the drain.

SUMMARY:

- Replace some of your conventional beauty care and household cleaning products with more natural alternatives, or try making your own products at home.

GUNK-FREE HABIT #21
Clean out the Clutter

> *"Clutter is a physical manifestation of fear that cripples our ability to grow."*- H.G. Chissel

Part of living gunk-free is de-cluttering and de-gunking your kitchen, home, car, office, and any other space that you visit on a daily basis. It is one thing to de-gunk your diet and your body, but it is just as important to de-gunk your environment. Clutter and excess "stuff" that we simply don't use or need, just adds to the feeling of overwhelm, and the inability to feel light and free.

Spend some time cleaning up and clearing out any clutter. The general rule is that if you have not used an item within one year, it is simply adding to unnecessary clutter and should be donated or recycled. Also, if you have not done so already, clear out any items in your kitchen that you are no longer going to consume. There is no need to keep old jars or bags of food that no longer serve your gunk-free lifestyle. You will be amazed at how light and energized you feel once you have purged unnecessary clutter in your home.

Don't look at cleaning up as one massive task. Tackle each section of the house, office, or kitchen in small increments. Even if you only clear out and organize a few drawers each day, you will quickly begin to feel the difference. When your living space is clean and healthy, you too will feel that way.

An organized space is a functional space, and therefore an organized kitchen is a functional kitchen. This means that it will be much easier and quicker to prepare healthy meals. An organized kitchen also makes it more inviting, so you are more likely to spend time playing around with new ingredients and getting creative with healthy meals.

Tips for Organizing Your Kitchen

- Store dry goods such as oatmeal, raw legumes, nuts, and seeds into glass or ceramic jars. Label the jars for easy identification.

- When transferring items from their original packaging into glass jars, or other storage containers, place a sticker with the expiration date on the container.
- Assign different drawers or bins for specific kitchen tools, such as measuring tools, spatulas, ladles, wooden spoons, etc., or use dividers in each drawer.
- Pre-wash and cut vegetables. Store them in divided BPA free containers in your fridge, or in the crisper drawer in your fridge.
- Be logical when organizing your kitchen
    - » Put the pots/pans by the stove
    - » Put baking sheets by the oven
    - » Put spices by the stove
    - » Store things close to where you use them. You do not want to be running all around the kitchen when trying to make dinner
- Organize your fridge/pantry and keep like items together:
    - » Crackers and snacks together
    - » Cereals and oatmeal together
    - » Pasta and rice together
    - » Legumes and dry grains together
    - » Natural sweeteners together
    - » Superfoods together
    - » Designate shelves or sections of your fridge for specific items. Have a section for drinks, leftovers, fruits, vegetables, oils, prepared foods, etc...
- Date leftovers so that you know when you made them and how long they are good for.
- Have a "garbage bowl" set up when preparing meals, where you can place all composting. This keeps you from running back and forth to the garbage. Simply use the "garbage bowl" during preparation, and empty it after.
- Keep your recipes organized. Keep a book or folder where you can organize your recipes.
- Use jars, baskets, and containers with labels to keep your pantry organized.

The 21-Day Gunk-Free Guide

ABOUT THE 21-DAY GUNK-FREE GUIDE

The 21-day gunk-free guide (beginning on page 156) is designed to get you started on your path to wellness in a simple, effective and painless way. The 21-day gunk-free guide introduces you to the healthy habits outlined in this book over the course of twenty-one days. It teaches you how to implement the gunk-free habits into your life in a step-by-step manner. It provides structure, by clearly defining what steps to take and in what order.

Getting started can be tough, and even though the gunk-free habits outlined in this book are simple to implement, following the twenty-one day guide helps to eliminate any guesswork. The twenty-one day guide provides you with daily tasks and checklists, which help to keep you on track.

Since this book is a "see-what-works-for-you-and-what-doesn't" type of book, it will be up to you to decide how many of the healthy habits you can, and want, to live with long-term. Even incorporating a few of the twenty-one recommendations long-term is better than none at all.

HOW TO FOLLOW THE GUIDE ON PAGE 156

On day one, implement the first habit to the best of your ability. On day two, add the second habit, while still following the habit from day one. The same goes for day three, where you will then have three habits to include that day. By day twenty-one, you will have implemented twenty-one healthy diet and lifestyle habits into your daily routine.

To make this program easy for you to follow, and for that added sense of accomplishment at the end of each day, there are "check it off" lists on page 167. These lists enable you to check off what you have done each day in order to track your progress.

POWER THROUGH

While you will begin to feel amazing after only a few short days, you may also experience some not-so-great feelings as you begin your gunk-free journey. Many people experience no physical symptoms or signs of withdrawal at all, however; some do. Those who experience symptoms such as headaches, fogginess, and fatigue are typically experiencing symptoms of withdrawal, since after all, we can become addicted to certain foods or substances over time. These symptoms are a sign that your body is doing its job of riding your system of refined sugars, artificial ingredients, and other chemical-filled substances. Those not-so-pleasant feelings do pass within a few days, and from then on you will only begin to feel refreshed and fabulous. Don't give up. Power through and you will see how truly amazing you can feel!

Initially you may experience cravings for sugar, alcohol, and caffeine (depending on how much of this you normally consume). But again, these feelings are just a reminder of how dependent your body has become. Breaking these habits and retraining your body to feel great without them is the ultimate goal.

Over the twenty-one days, you will slowly abstain from caffeine, alcohol, refined sugar, and processed foods, and load yourself full of healthy, natural and nourishing foods. You will also incorporate healthy lifestyle and basic cleansing practices into your daily routine that will work to clean out your digestive system and other major organs of detoxification. Essentially, you are giving your body a much needed and well-deserved break.

PREPARATION – BEFORE YOU BEGIN YOUR 21-DAY JOURNEY

BEFORE USING THE 21-DAY GUNK-FREE GUIDE, MAKE SURE TO READ THE INTRODUCTION SECTION OF THIS BOOK ON PAGES xxiii-21.

WEEK 1 – DE-GUNK YOUR DIET

Day 1 – Set Realistic Goals

It is important to set realistic goals. Using the gunk-free goal-planning sheet provided on page 24, take some time today to think about what you want to achieve (both with this program and in your life in general). Your goals do not have to be set to be achieved within twenty-one days (although it is a good idea to set at least one big goal that you would like to achieve over the course of your twenty-one day journey). Instead, they can be goals that you set to achieve over a longer period of time.

- Read pages 23-25 -

Day 2 - Cut the Coffee and Cola and Sip on Some Tea

For coffee drinkers: Reduce your intake of coffee. Slowly reduce the amount of coffee you consume to avoid withdrawal symptoms. If you normally drink three coffees per day, reduce to two for a few days, then to one, then to none. Or, reduce the size of your cup each day, having less and days go on.

For non-coffee drinkers: Increase your intake of green or herbal teas, or try including maca into your smoothies.

For everyone: Completely eliminate soda from your diet.

- Read pages 26-34 -

Day 3 – Lose the Booze

Eliminate alcohol from your diet. If you consume alcohol on a regular basis, challenge yourself to eliminate it completely over the course of your gunk-free journey. If you do not consume alcohol, continue focusing on following the recommendations from days one and two. Continue to enjoy delicious gunk-free foods and eliminate the "gunk-filled" foods.

- Read pages 35-36 -

Day 4 – Replace Refined Sugar and Get More Whole Grains

Replace all refined sugar (including products made with it) with healthier, natural alternatives. Go completely refined sugar-free for the duration of your 21-day journey.

Say goodbye to cakes, cookies, breads and pastas made with refined flour, and say hello to whole grains! Eliminate all "white" products from your diet and replace them with nourishing whole grains and other fiber-rich complex carbohydrates. Consume between 25-40 grams of fiber each day.

- Read pages 37-56 -

Day 5 – No More Moo

Dairy is a common allergen, contributes to digestive upset, is highly inflammatory, and mucus forming. In order to effectively de-gunk your body, it is best to avoid dairy completely for the duration of your 21-day journey.

This means avoiding cow's milk, cheese, butter, cream, sour cream, margarine, and ice cream, and any products containing dairy.

- Read pages 57-65 -

Day 6 – Time to Veg

Consume a variety of colorful fruits and vegetables. Try to incorporate seven to ten servings of fruits and vegetables into your daily diet. Try to incorporate leafy green vegetables into each meal.

- Read pages 80-87 -

Day 7 – Eat Clean, Lean Protein and Healthy Fat

<u>Protein</u>

Consume clean protein from organic, grass-fed, free-range meats. Includes: lean meats, fish (wild caught), poultry, and eggs, as well as legumes, nuts and seeds.

Vegan Options (Not just for vegans!)

Includes, tempeh (fermented soy), sprouted tofu, legumes (chickpeas, lentils, etc.,), nuts, seeds, and green vegetables.

<u>Fat</u>

Include "good" fats into your diet, while making sure to strictly avoid "bad" fats. Try to include a healthy fat at each meal. Good fats include: flax seeds, chia seeds, sunflower seeds, sesame seeds, beans, avocado, coconut oil, olive oil, nuts and fatty fish (salmon, tuna, mackerel, herring, cod, trout).

Avoid: High fat meats (beef, pork), cheese, ice cream, commercially baked cookies, muffins, and cakes, anything that contains trans fat, margarine, vegetable shortening, and fried foods.

- Read pages 66-79 -

WEEK 2 – DE-GUNK YOUR BODY

Day 8 – Drink More Water and Squeeze Some Lemon + Optional Juicing

Add the juice of half a fresh lemon to a glass of room temperature (or warm) water each morning (on an empty stomach before breakfast).

Drink at least eight glasses of fresh, pure, clean water everyday. This is one of the best ways to detoxify our bodies, speed up metabolism, and prevent dehydration.

Optional: Incorporate a fresh, homemade vegetable/fruit juice into your daily diet. Consume on an empty stomach if possible. Best to have in the morning before breakfast. Juice three vegetables for every one fruit. Can have juice in place of lemon water, if lemon is included in your juice.

-Read pages 88-100 -

Day 9 – Say Yes to Superfoods

Include at least one (or more) superfoods into your daily diet. Do not stick to the same superfoods everyday. Try to include each of the superfoods listed at least once throughout your gunk-free journey.

- Read pages 101-111 -

Day 10 – Exercise

Get at least 20-30 minutes of physical exercise each day. Run, walk, skip, swim, lift weights, or even dance in your room. Whatever it is, just keep your body moving!

- Read pages 112-115 -

Day 11 – Sip on A Smoothie

Consume a healthy smoothie daily as a snack, before or after a workout, or as part of a healthy breakfast.

- Read pages 116-120 -

Day 12 – Make Friends with Probiotics

Consume probiotic-rich foods and/or supplement with a high quality probiotic supplement daily, in order to maintain a healthy gut.

- Read pages 121-125 -

Day 13 – Add Some Spice and Soothe with Some Parsley and Ginger Tea

Add a variety of herbs and spices to your food for a more fragrant, nutrient-rich meal. Make sure to include at least one herb or spice at each meal. Includes: garlic, ginger, parsley, turmeric and cinnamon.

Drink ¼ cup of homemade parsley and ginger tea each morning (or at a time that is convenient for you).

- Read pages 126-130 -

Day 14 – Brush Your Skin, Dry

Practice dry skin brushing on a daily basis (or as often as possible). This helps to detoxify the body and remove impurities from the outside in.

- Read pages 131-132 -

WEEK 3 – DE-GUNK YOUR LIFE

Day 15 – Take It All In

Think of today as a day off (sort of). There are no NEW habits today, but instead, today is a chance to reflect on what you have done (or not done) thus far.

It is important to take a moment to stop and reflect. Today is really a chance to check in with yourself to see how you are doing/feeling so far on your journey to health and wellness. What healthy changes have you made? What are some things you are still working on? How are you feeling? What has been your biggest accomplishment so far?

We all live busy lives, and often forget to take the time to reflect. We often look at how far we have to go, and neglect to see how far we have already come. Today, take the time to cheer for the steps you have already taken, and try to include some of the ones that you have not tried thus far.

It is a good idea to re-read some of the previous gunk-free habits – you may have missed something or forgotten about them by now. You may also find that you want to make changes, add, or adjust to what you have already done and see if there is anything new you might want to try.

Today's big goal: Incorporate all of the fourteen recommendations provided in this guide thus far. It can be challenging to incorporate every habit each day, so if you have not yet done so, try doing it today, and see how it goes.

You should be very proud of your accomplishments so far. Go ahead, toot your own horn and give yourself a pat on the back - you deserve it!

Day 16 – Get Better Sleep

Proper sleep is essential in order to restore our bodies and refresh our minds.

When we sleep, immune enhancing chemicals are released which help to protect our immune system and improve overall health. Without adequate sleep, our natural killer cells (cells which destroy germs) do not function optimally.

It is important to get 6-8 hours of sleep per night. The quality of sleep had is just as important as the amount of time slept. Sleeping from one o'clock am to nine o'clock am is not thought to be as restorative as sleeping from ten o'clock pm to six o'clock am.

So tonight, and over the course of your gunk-free journey (and hopefully even after that), try to get to bed by ten o'clock pm.

- Read pages 134-135 -

Day 17 - De-Gunk Your Mind and Unwind

You time is one of the most important things that you can do for yourself, your health, and your stress levels. All you have to do is schedule at least twenty minutes each day just for YOU. This time is for you to relax and do what you enjoy, away from everyone and everything else that might need or want your attention. Read, practice yoga, walk around the block, meditate, take a bath or get a massage. Just do whatever it is that you like to do, without distraction. This time is so incredibly important as it enables you to check in with yourself and unwind. You will find that just twenty minutes a day makes a huge difference.

- Read pages 137-140 -

Day 18 - Undress Your Stress

Incorporate some vitamin B and magnesium rich foods into your diet. This will help to calm and relax your adrenal glands and combat stress.

By now, you have likely incorporated many of these foods into your daily diet, however today is a chance for you to up your intake of them, or try some new items.

- **Vitamin B rich foods:** Beans, liver, wheat bran, bananas, oats, turkey, avocado, salmon, lentils, spinach, turnip greens, eggs, and whole grains.

- **Magnesium rich foods**: Bananas, figs, oat bran, brown rice, almonds, beans, pumpkin seeds, spinach.

* Can also supplement with B vitamins and magnesium. Follow instructions on bottle.

- Read pages 135 and 137 -

Day 19 – Go Chemical-Free

De-gunk your beauty care products and household cleaners. Avoid products with harsh chemicals and choose products made with natural ingredients. Another great option is to make them yourself with nourishing, healing ingredients.

- Read pages 142-149 -

Day 20 – Clean Out the Clutter

Part of living gunk-free is de-cluttering and de-gunking your home, car, office, and any other space that you visit on a daily basis. It is one thing to de-gunk your diet and your body, but it is just as important to de-gunk your environment. Take some time today to clean up and clear out any clutter. The general rule is that if you have not used an item within one year, it is simply adding to unnecessary clutter and should be donated or recycled. Also, if you have not done so already, clear out any items in your kitchen cupboards that no longer serve your gunk-free lifestyle. You will be amazed at how light and gunk-free you feel once you have purged unnecessary clutter in your home.

- Read pages 150-151 -

Day 21 – Do A Happy Dance!

Congratulations! You have made it to day 21. Do a little happy dance. You have made some amazing, beneficial, healthy changes and you should be very proud of yourself!

Today, take everything you have learned and implemented so far, and challenge yourself to include every single one of those changes into your routine today. Let's finish this off with a bang!

Go through today's check it off list and plan your day around including all of these items into your routine at some point today. Now, this may not be physically possible for you today, depending on your schedule, so do as much as you can – challenge yourself to do even a little bit more than you think you can.

At this point, you have a long list of healthy, cleansing, and nourishing recommendations that you can choose to carry with you long-term or leave behind as a fond memory of your gunk-free journey. It is recommended however, that you continue following these recommendations for at least another week, on your own, at your own pace. Some recommendations that were made in the second half of this guide are still fairly new to you, so giving yourself another week or so to become more comfortable with them is a good idea.

After the 21 Days – Living Gunk-Free Long-Term

- If you choose, you can begin to reintroduce dairy and see how you feel. If you notice that you become congested or suffer from digestive upset, adopting a dairy-free lifestyle long-term is recommended.
- Continue to consume fresh fruits and vegetables, lean protein, healthy fats, complex carbohydrates, and between 25-40 grams of fiber each day.
- Continue to avoid refined sugar and use healthier sugar alternatives.
- Continue to avoid coffee and consume herbal teas and/or coffee alternatives. Or, consume organic coffee on an occasional basis.
- Continue to avoid alcohol, or enjoy it on an occasional basis.
- Continue to drink at least eight glasses of water each day.
- Continue to consume lemon water each morning.

- Include a fresh juice or smoothie into your daily diet, or even a few times per week.
- Consume superfoods on a regular basis.
- Exercise at least three times per week – break a sweat!
- Consume probiotic-rich foods or supplement with a high quality probiotic for maintenance long-term.
- Use a variety of spices in your cooking and consume a parsley and ginger tea when desired.
- Perform dry skin brushing a few times per week to continue detoxifying your body.
- Get between six to eight hours of sleep every night.
- Go chemical-free as much as possible.
- Take time every day, or at least every week, for YOU time.
- Keep your home and kitchen clutter-free, and do a big de-cluttering every four to six months.

Continue to set realistic goals and work to achieve them. Continue to implement many or all of the healthy habits in this book long-term and stick to the ones that suit you best.

Get The Gunk Out "Check It Off" Lists

Day 1

☐ Set realistic goals

Day 2

☐ Set realistic goals
☐ Cut the coffee and cola and sip on some tea

Day 3

☐ Set realistic goals
☐ Cut the coffee and cola and sip on some tea
☐ No alcohol

Day 4

☐ Set realistic goals
☐ Cut the coffee and cola and sip on some tea
☐ No alcohol
☐ No refined sugar and get more whole grains

Day 5

☐ Set realistic goals
☐ Cut the coffee and cola and sip on some tea
☐ No alcohol
☐ No refined sugar and get more whole grains
☐ No dairy

Day 6

☐ Set realistic goals
☐ Cut the coffee and cola and sip on some tea
☐ No alcohol
☐ No refined sugar and get more whole grains
☐ No dairy
☐ Eat more vegetables and fruit

Day 7
- ☐ Set realistic goals
- ☐ Cut the coffee and cola and sip on some tea
- ☐ No alcohol
- ☐ No refined sugar and get more whole grains
- ☐ No dairy
- ☐ Eat more vegetables and fruit
- ☐ Eat clean, lean protein and healthy fat

Day 8
- ☐ Set realistic goals
- ☐ Cut the coffee and cola and sip on some tea
- ☐ No alcohol
- ☐ No refined sugar and get more whole grains
- ☐ No dairy
- ☐ Eat more vegetables and fruit
- ☐ Eat clean, lean protein and healthy fat
- ☐ Drink lots of water & squeeze some lemon and/or make a fresh juice

Day 9
- ☐ Set realistic goals
- ☐ Cut the coffee and cola and sip on some tea
- ☐ No alcohol
- ☐ No refined sugar and get more whole grains
- ☐ No dairy
- ☐ Eat more vegetables and fruit
- ☐ Eat clean, lean protein and healthy fat
- ☐ Drink lots of water & squeeze some lemon and/or make a fresh juice
- ☐ Eat a variety of superfoods

Day 10
- ☐ Set realistic goals
- ☐ Cut the coffee and cola and sip on some tea
- ☐ No alcohol
- ☐ No refined sugar and get more whole grains
- ☐ No dairy
- ☐ Eat more vegetables and fruit
- ☐ Eat clean, lean protein and healthy fat
- ☐ Drink lots of water & squeeze some lemon and/or make a fresh juice
- ☐ Eat a variety of superfoods
- ☐ Exercise

Day 11
- [ ] Set realistic goals
- [ ] Cut the coffee and cola and sip on some tea
- [ ] No alcohol
- [ ] No refined sugar and get more whole grains
- [ ] No dairy
- [ ] Eat more vegetables and fruit
- [ ] Eat clean, lean protein and healthy fat
- [ ] Drink lots of water & squeeze some lemon and/or make a fresh juice
- [ ] Eat a variety of superfoods
- [ ] Exercise
- [ ] Make a smoothie

Day 12
- [ ] Set realistic goals
- [ ] Cut the coffee and cola and sip on some tea
- [ ] No alcohol
- [ ] No refined sugar and get more whole grains
- [ ] No dairy
- [ ] Eat more vegetables and fruit
- [ ] Eat clean, lean protein and healthy fat
- [ ] Drink lots of water & squeeze some lemon and/or make a fresh juice
- [ ] Eat a variety of superfoods
- [ ] Exercise
- [ ] Make a smoothie
- [ ] Probiotics

Day 13
- [ ] Set realistic goals
- [ ] Cut the coffee and cola and sip on some tea
- [ ] No alcohol
- [ ] No refined sugar and get more whole grains
- [ ] No dairy
- [ ] Eat more vegetables and fruit
- [ ] Eat clean, lean protein and healthy fat
- [ ] Drink lots of water & squeeze some lemon and/or make a fresh juice
- [ ] Eat a variety of superfoods
- [ ] Exercise
- [ ] Make a smoothie
- [ ] Probiotics
- [ ] Include spices into your diet and drink parsley and ginger tea

Day 14
- [ ] Set realistic goals
- [ ] Cut the coffee and cola and sip on some tea
- [ ] No alcohol
- [ ] No refined sugar and get more whole grains
- [ ] No dairy
- [ ] Eat more vegetables and fruit
- [ ] Eat clean, lean protein and healthy fat
- [ ] Drink lots of water & squeeze some lemon and/or make a fresh juice
- [ ] Eat a variety of superfoods
- [ ] Exercise
- [ ] Make a smoothie
- [ ] Probiotics
- [ ] Include spices into your diet and drink parsley and ginger tea
- [ ] Dry skin brushing

Day 15
- [ ] Set realistic goals
- [ ] Cut the coffee and cola and sip on some tea
- [ ] No alcohol
- [ ] No refined sugar and get more whole grains
- [ ] No dairy
- [ ] Eat more vegetables and fruit
- [ ] Eat clean, lean protein and healthy fat
- [ ] Drink lots of water & squeeze some lemon and/or make a fresh juice
- [ ] Eat a variety of superfoods
- [ ] Exercise
- [ ] Make a smoothie
- [ ] Probiotics
- [ ] Include spices into your diet and drink parsley and ginger tea
- [ ] Dry skin brushing
- [ ] Check in with yourself

Day 16
- [ ] Set realistic goals
- [ ] Cut the coffee and cola and sip on some tea
- [ ] No alcohol
- [ ] No refined sugar and get more whole grains
- [ ] No dairy
- [ ] Eat more vegetables and fruit
- [ ] Eat clean, lean protein and healthy fat
- [ ] Drink lots of water & squeeze some lemon and/or make a fresh juice
- [ ] Eat a variety of superfoods

- ☐ Exercise
- ☐ Make a smoothie
- ☐ Probiotics
- ☐ Include spices into your diet and drink parsley and ginger tea
- ☐ Dry skin brushing
- ☐ Check in with yourself
- ☐ Sleep well (between 6-8 hours)

Day 17

- ☐ Set realistic goals
- ☐ Cut the coffee and cola and sip on some tea
- ☐ No alcohol
- ☐ No refined sugar and get more whole grains
- ☐ No dairy
- ☐ Eat more vegetables and fruit
- ☐ Eat clean, lean protein and healthy fat
- ☐ Drink lots of water & squeeze some lemon and/or make a fresh juice
- ☐ Eat a variety of superfoods
- ☐ Exercise
- ☐ Make a smoothie
- ☐ Probiotics
- ☐ Include spices into your diet and drink parsley and ginger tea
- ☐ Dry skin brushing
- ☐ Check in with yourself
- ☐ Sleep well (between 6-8 hours)
- ☐ Make YOU time – De-gunk your mind and unwind

Day 18

- ☐ Set realistic goals
- ☐ Cut the coffee and cola and sip on some tea
- ☐ No alcohol
- ☐ No refined sugar and get more whole grains
- ☐ No dairy
- ☐ Eat more vegetables and fruit
- ☐ Eat clean, lean protein and healthy fat
- ☐ Drink lots of water & squeeze some lemon and/or make a fresh juice
- ☐ Eat a variety of superfoods
- ☐ Exercise
- ☐ Make a smoothie
- ☐ Probiotics
- ☐ Include spices into your diet and drink parsley and ginger tea

- ☐ Dry skin brushing
- ☐ Check in with yourself
- ☐ Sleep well (between 6-8 hours)
- ☐ Make YOU time – De-gunk your mind and unwind
- ☐ Vitamin B and magnesium-rich foods

Day 19

- ☐ Set realistic goals
- ☐ Cut the coffee and cola and sip on some tea
- ☐ No alcohol
- ☐ No refined sugar and get more whole grains
- ☐ No dairy
- ☐ Eat more vegetables and fruit
- ☐ Eat clean, lean protein and healthy fat
- ☐ Drink lots of water & squeeze some lemon and/or make a fresh juice
- ☐ Eat a variety of superfoods
- ☐ Exercise
- ☐ Make a smoothie
- ☐ Probiotics
- ☐ Include spices into your diet and drink parsley and ginger tea
- ☐ Dry skin brushing
- ☐ Check in with yourself
- ☐ Sleep well (between 6-8 hours)
- ☐ Make YOU time – De-gunk your mind and unwind
- ☐ Vitamin B and magnesium-rich foods
- ☐ Go chemical-free

Day 20

- ☐ Set realistic goals
- ☐ Cut the coffee and cola and sip on some tea
- ☐ No alcohol
- ☐ No refined sugar and get more whole grains
- ☐ No dairy
- ☐ Eat more vegetables and fruit
- ☐ Eat clean, lean protein and healthy fat
- ☐ Drink lots of water & squeeze some lemon and/or make a fresh juice
- ☐ Eat a variety of superfoods
- ☐ Exercise

- ☐ Make a smoothie
- ☐ Probiotics
- ☐ Include spices into your diet and drink parsley and ginger tea
- ☐ Dry skin brushing
- ☐ Check in with yourself
- ☐ Sleep well (between 6-8 hours)
- ☐ Make YOU time – De-gunk your mind and unwind
- ☐ Vitamin B and magnesium-rich foods
- ☐ Go chemical-free
- ☐ Clean out the clutter

Day 21
- ☐ Set realistic goals
- ☐ Cut the coffee and cola and sip on some tea
- ☐ No alcohol
- ☐ No refined sugar and get more whole grains
- ☐ No dairy
- ☐ Eat more vegetables and fruit
- ☐ Eat clean, lean protein and healthy fat
- ☐ Drink lots of water & squeeze some lemon and/or make a fresh juice
- ☐ Eat a variety of superfoods
- ☐ Exercise
- ☐ Make a smoothie
- ☐ Probiotics
- ☐ Include spices into your diet and drink parsley and ginger tea
- ☐ Dry skin brushing
- ☐ Check in with yourself
- ☐ Sleep well (between 6-8 hours)
- ☐ Make YOU time – De-gunk your mind and unwind
- ☐ Vitamin B and magnesium-rich foods
- ☐ Go chemical-free
- ☐ Clean out the clutter
- ☐ Do a happy dance!

For printable checklists for long-term use, visit www.shannonkadlovski.com

**SIMPLE AND DELICIOUS
GUNK-FREE RECIPES**

Simple And Delicious Gunk-Free Recipes

See contents page for a complete list of recipes. See page 10 for a 7-day menu with additional meal ideas and recipes.

Whole Grain French Toast

Ingredients

2 slices whole grain bread
2 egg whites (or one egg white/one whole egg)
¼ tsp. cinnamon
½ banana
¼ cup fresh berries or other fruit (apple, peach, etc.)
pure maple syrup (to be drizzled on top)
1 tbsp. chia seeds or ground flax seeds
handful of nuts or 1 tbsp. nut or seed butter (optional)

Instructions

- Beat eggs in a small bowl
- Dip both slices of bread in egg and coat evenly
- Sprinkle with cinnamon
- Add some grape seed oil or coconut oil to your pan and turn heat to medium

- Place bread in pan. Cook 2 minutes on one side, flip and cook 2 minutes on the other. Should be golden brown before removing from pan.
- Top French toast with bananas and other fruit, drizzle with pure maple syrup and add some chia seeds or ground flax seeds.
- Optional - Can top with nuts or nut/seed butter

Gluten-Free Pancakes

Ingredients

1 banana
2 egg whites
¼ cup brown rice flour or coconut flour or chickpea flour (or other gluten-free flour)
1 tbsp. ground flax seed
1 tbsp. dried shredded coconut

Top pancakes with 1 tbsp. sunflower seed butter or other nut/seed butter with ¼ cup fresh berries or 1-2 tbsp. pure maple syrup with ¼ cup fresh berries

Instructions

- Combine all ingredients in a bowl
- Lightly oil a stainless steel pan with coconut oil or grape seed oil
- Drop batter into pan by the spoonful
- Once batter starts to bubble, flip pancake and cook the other side
- Pancakes are ready when the top has hardened to a golden brown

Morning Muesli

This should be made the night before you wish to consume it, as an overnight soaking of the ingredients is recommended. You can make a large batch and keep it in the fridge to be consumed as a ready-to-go breakfast during the week.

Ingredients

1 cups of rolled oats
1 cup of quinoa flakes
½ cup unsulphured raisins
½ cup nuts and seeds (almonds, walnuts, sunflower seeds)
¼ cup unsweetened shredded coconut
Coconut milk (or other milk alternative) – enough to cover the contents in the bowl
1 tsp. ground cinnamon

Toppings to add before eating (as many as you like)

Handful cacao nibs
1 tbsp. chia seeds or ground flax seeds
1 tsp. raw honey or pure maple syrup
1 tbsp. goji berries
Extra cinnamon
Fresh fruit (apple, berries, peaches, etc.,)

Instructions

- Combine all ingredients (except toppings), in a large bowl. Pour in the coconut milk or other milk alternative (should just cover the contents in the bowl)
- Place the bowl in the refrigerator and let it rest overnight
- Right before eating, add in your favourite toppings

* Store in an airtight container for up to 3 days.

Heavenly Chocolate Protein Smoothie

> 2 cups brown rice milk
> 1 tbsp. sunflower seed butter
> 1 tsp. manuka honey
> 1 tbsp. date paste or 5 pitted dates
> 1 tbsp. chia seeds
> 1 scoop or 2 tbsp. protein powder
> 2 tbsp. cocoa powder or raw cacao powder
> 1 cup mixed berries and mango (frozen)
> 1 cup of kale
>
> * Toss all ingredients into a blender and blend until smooth and creamy

Scrumptious Superfood Smoothie

> 1 cup water or coconut water
> 1 scoop protein powder (or 2 tbsp. if it doesn't come with a scoop)
> 1 tbsp. chia seeds
> 1 tsp. matcha green tea powder
> 1 tsp. fish oil
> 1 tsp. spirulina powder
> ½ cup fresh blueberries
>
> * Toss all of the ingredients into a blender and blend until smooth and creamy

The Energizer Smoothie

> 1 cup coconut water (can use regular water or milk alternative)
> 1 tsp. maca
> 1 tsp. matcha green tea powder
> 2 tbsp. protein powder
> handful of spinach
> 1/4 avocado
> 1/4 cup blueberries
> ½ tbsp. chia seeds
> 1 tsp. raw honey
> * Toss all of the ingredients into a blender and blend until smooth and creamy

Pumpkin Spice Smoothie

> 1 cup almond milk
> ½ cup pumpkin puree (or cooked sweet potato)
> ½ of a banana
> 1 tsp. cinnamon
> pinch nutmeg
> 2 tbsp. protein powder (plain or vanilla)
> 1 tbsp. pure maple syrup
> * Toss all of the ingredients into a blender and blend until smooth and creamy

Coco-Nutty Smoothie (can be made nut-free)

½ cup coconut milk
½ cup coconut water
¼ cup fresh coconut or dried coconut
2 tbsp. natural nut or seed butter
1 tbsp. chia seeds
1 tbsp. pure maple syrup
* Toss all of the ingredients into a blender and blend until smooth and creamy

DIPS/SPREADS/SAUCES

Hearty Hummus

Ingredients

1 cup dry chickpeas (use entire batch once cooked) or 2 ½ cans chickpeas
4 cups water (to cook dry chickpeas) – no water needed for canned chickpeas
¼ cup tahini
½ - 1 tsp. sea salt
1 clove garlic (can add more garlic to taste)
1/3 cup fresh squeezed lemon

<u>Instructions using dry chickpeas</u>
- Soak chickpeas in water overnight
- Strain and rinse well
- Add water and chickpeas to pot and bring to a boil
- Cover and simmer using low heat for 1-2 hours

- Place cooked chickpeas into blender or food processor (saving some of the water in the pot to add back if hummus is too thick)
- Add the rest of the ingredients and blend/process until smooth
- Scoop hummus into a bowl. Drizzle with some olive oil on top and sprinkle with paprika.

<u>Instructions using caned chickpeas</u>
- Process the chickpeas in a blender or food processor with the rest of the ingredients. (If it is too thick add some water).
- Scoop hummus into a bowl.
- Drizzle some olive oil on top and sprinkle with paprika.

Serve with whole grain crackers or homemade honey sesame crackers (page 204) and/or fresh veggies (cucumber, celery, peppers and carrots).

Avocado and Goat Cheese Dip

Ingredients

2 ripe avocados
2 tbsp. goat cheese – crumbled
2 cloves garlic – crushed
¼ cup parsley – chopped
½ tsp. sea salt
¼ tsp. black pepper (or to taste)
1 lime – freshly squeezed

<u>Instructions</u>
- Mash avocados in a bowl using a fork
- Add the rest of the ingredients and combine well (can also use a food processor)

* Serve with homemade crackers (page 204) or any whole grain or gluten-free cracker. Can also serve with fresh vegetables or on bread as part of a sandwich.

Simple Salsa

Ingredients

3 tomatoes – chopped
1 tbsp. tomato paste (optional)
1 lime – juiced
½ tbsp. olive oil
1-2 green onions – chopped
½ cup cilantro or parsley – chopped
½ cup green bell pepper – chopped
* Can add chopped jalapeno peppers for a spicier salsa

Instructions

- Combine all ingredients into a bowl and serve

Pineapple Sauce

Ingredients

1 cup pineapple juice (freshly juiced if possible or one without added sugar)
1/3 cup water
3 tbsp. rice vinegar or balsamic vinegar
1 tbsp. Braggs or Tamari soy sauce
1/4 cup sucanat (can use ¼ cup maple syrup instead)
1/2 tsp. salt
1 tbsp. chia seeds or ground flax
½ - 1 cup fresh pineapple chunks (optional)

Instructions

- Place chia or ground flax seeds into ¼ cup water and allow it to thicken. It will form a gel.
- Combine all ingredients into a saucepan and heat over low/medium for 10-15 minutes or until it begins to thicken.

Note:

You can use 4-5 tsp. arrowroot or brown rice flour in place of the flax or chia. Mix arrowroot or brown rice flour with ¼ cup water to form a paste before adding it to the recipe. If you add it directly to the sauce without creating a paste, it can become lumpy.

Can be used for a baked chicken recipe: Pour sauce on top of chicken and bake at 350 degrees for 20-25 minutes.

Can be used for stir-fry, meatballs, or to marinate tempeh.

Garlic Parsley Sauce (as a marinade or on top of chicken/fish/pasta)

Ingredients

3 cloves fresh garlic – minced
1 cup chopped fresh parsley
2 tbsp. apple cider vinegar
1 tbsp. chopped onion
½ cup extra virgin olive oil
1/8 tsp. sea salt
1/8 tsp. chili powder

Instructions

- Place ingredients into a hand blender or food processor and pulse until desired consistency.
- Use as a marinade or on top of chicken/fish/pasta or any other dish.
- Store in the refrigerator for up to 3 days.

Creamy Chocolate Hazelnut Spread

Ingredients

2 cups raw hazelnuts (240g)
1 tbsp. pure vanilla extract
1/4 cup cocoa powder or 6 ounces pure dark chocolate
¼ cup + 3 tbsp. pure maple syrup or honey OR ½ cup coconut sugar
1/4 tsp. sea salt
1/2 cup milk alternative (coconut milk, almond milk, rice milk, hemp milk)

Instructions

- Place raw hazelnuts on a baking sheet and roast for 10-15 minutes at 400 F.
- Remove from oven and place hazelnuts onto a towel, rubbing them together to remove the skin.
- If using pure dark chocolate, melt the chocolate using a double boiler (boil a pot of water over high heat. Place chocolate in a stainless steel bowl and place overtop of the water to be melted.
- In a food processor or high-speed blender, combine the nuts until creamy.
- Add in vanilla, cocoa powder or melted chocolate, sweetener of choice, salt and milk alternative of choice. Blend until smooth and creamy.
- Store the chocolate hazelnut spread in a mason jar or other glass jar, in the refrigerator, for up to 2 weeks.

Tip: Spread some chocolate hazelnut goodness on whole grain toast and top with 1 tsp. ground flax seeds or chia seeds and sliced banana.

MAINS

Hearty Turkey Chili – serves 4-6 people

Ingredients

1 package lean ground turkey
1 large can of crushed or diced tomatoes (organic)
1 can of tomato paste (organic)
Fresh garlic or garlic salt
Sea salt (can add kelp powder as well)
1 tsp. dried basil
1 tsp. dried oregano
Fresh vegetables of your choice (zucchini, mushrooms, onions, peppers, broccoli, etc...)
1 cup chickpeas or kidney beans (or both)

Instructions

- Cook ground turkey over medium heat in a pan on the stove (strain the excess juice once cooked)
- Cook veggies in a wok with water or steam them in water until they start to soften (do not over cook vegetables)
- Place 1 can of tomatoes and 1 can of tomato paste in a pot and cook on low
- Add salt, basil, oregano, and garlic to sauce
- Add beans to sauce and simmer for 15-20 mins
- Add veggies and ground turkey to sauce and combine all ingredients
- Serve hot

Tasty Tamari Tempeh

<u>Marinade Ingredients (this marinade can be used on chicken, fish or pasta as well)</u>

> ¼ cup Tamari (or other wheat-free soy sauce)
> 2 tbsp. pure maple syrup
> 2 tsp. olive oil
> 1 tbsp. chopped onion
> 1-2 cloves chopped garlic

<u>Instructions</u>

- Thaw 1 block of tempeh
- Place into glass dish (or oven friendly dish) and pour marinade over top
- Marinade in fridge for 2 hours (if time permits)
- Bake in the oven at 350°F for 30 minutes (covered)
- Remove from oven and cut tempeh into cubes, strips, or bite sized pieces

Tempeh can be added to quinoa salad, stir-fry, tempeh-kebabs, or eaten on it's own with a side salad, mashed sweet potatoes and cooked veggies.

Quinoa Veggie Burgers

* Makes 6-8 patties

Ingredients

1 ½ cups cooked quinoa
½ cup cooked (or canned) chickpeas – mashed, using 2-3 tbsp. water
¼ cup finely chopped zucchini and mushrooms (or vegetables of choice)
¼ cup rolled oats
1 tbsp. chopped onion
1 tbsp. olive oil
1 tbsp. Braggs or Tamari
1 clove fresh garlic or ½ tsp. garlic powder
¼ cup brown rice flour or chickpea flour (or other gluten-free flour)
1 tsp. dried basil
1 tsp. dried oregano
½ tsp. sea salt
½ tsp. black pepper

Instructions

- Combine all ingredients in a large bowl or food processor
- Allow the mixture to sit (in refrigerator) for one hour (if possible) – this allows the patties to form better
- Form mixture into patties (makes 6-8)
- Cook in a cast iron skillet, on stovetop, over medium heat, for 5 minutes on each side (or until browned). Cook with a little bit of grape seed oil in the pan
- Serve with whole grain or gluten-free buns or without a bun (on top of lettuce and vegetables of your choice)

Baked Chicken (or Turkey) Meatballs - makes 20-24 meatballs

Ingredients

2 pounds lean ground turkey or chicken
1/2 cup chopped basil or parsley
3 garlic cloves - minced
1 tsp. sea salt
¼ teaspoon black pepper
1/2 cup spelt (or gluten-free) breadcrumbs
2 eggs or ½ cup chia gel (page 75)

Sauce

4 cups canned, crushed tomatoes
1 clove garlic - crushed
1/2 tsp. sea salt
black pepper to taste
1 tsp. fresh or dried basil
1 tsp. fresh or dried parsley

Instructions

- Preheat oven to 450°F
- Grease a baking dish with grape seed oil
- Combine all ingredients into a mixing bowl and mix by hand
- Roll mixture into medium sized balls
- Place meatballs into baking dish, lining them up in rows
- Bake for 20-25 minutes or until meatballs are fully cooked through
- Place all sauce ingredients into a small pot and cook on low/medium heat
- Place meatballs and sauce into large serving bowl and serve hot

Tempeh Lettuce Wraps

Ingredients

1 head of lettuce – romaine or cabbage
1 cup cooked brown rice noodles or buckwheat noodles
½ bell pepper – sliced into strips
5 mushrooms – sliced into strips
¼ purple onion – sliced into strips
¼ zucchini – sliced into strips
2 cups bean sprouts
½ - 1 cup cooked tempeh (page 188) – sliced into strips

Sauce

¼ cup Tamari or Braggs soy sauce
2 tbsp. raw honey
1 clove fresh crushed garlic
1 tbsp. fresh dill

Instructions

- Cook brown rice noodles or buckwheat noodles in a pot of boiling water until soft
- Drain liquid from pot and rinse with cold water. Set aside
- Combine sauce ingredients into small bowl
- Slice vegetables and steam them on or cook on medium heat in a wok with some grape seed oil or water
- Add in bean sprouts for the last 2-3 minutes of cook-time
- Bake tempeh (see page 188 for marinade and cooking instructions)
- Place cooked vegetables, noodles and tempeh into a large bowl and pour sauce on top. Mix together

- Using individual pieces of lettuce as your shell, fill each full leaf of lettuce with the vegetable, noodle and tempeh mixture. Fill the center, but leave room around the edges to roll the lettuce into a wrap
- Wrap each piece of lettuce with the delicious mixture and enjoy!

Options:

- Can omit the noodles and replace with rice, or nothing at all
- Can replace tempeh with cooked chicken
- Can top with chopped nuts or seeds

Maple Miso Glazed Salmon

Ingredients

¼ cup pure maple syrup (or other wheat-free soy sauce)
1 tbsp. red miso (or 2 tbsp. wheat-free soy sauce)
1 tbsp. olive oil
1 tbsp. chopped onion
1 tbsp. freshly grated ginger
pinch of sea salt
2 7oz salmon fillets

Instructions

- In a small bowl, combine miso, maple syrup, olive oil, chopped onion, and ginger. Set aside
- Sprinkle sea salt on top of salmon

Baking instructions

- Place salmon in a glass baking dish and pour mixture over top
- Allow the salmon to marinate in the fridge for 30 minutes
- Bake at 425°F for 12 minutes

Stovetop instructions

- Coat a cast iron or stainless steel skillet with grape seed oil and turn heat to medium

- Allow the skillet to heat up (drop a few drops of water into the pan, if it sizzles, it's hot enough)
- Pour half of the miso/maple mixture on top of the salmon and place salmon into the skillet, skin side up. Cook for 4 minutes over medium heat
- Flip salmon over using a spatula and pour the rest of the mixture overtop. Cook for another 4-5 minutes, until cooked through
- Remove from pan and serve

SALADS & VEGETABLES

Tempeh & Quinoa Salad

Note: This recipe includes tamari tempeh, however, you can replace the tempeh with chickpeas, fresh turkey, or chicken.

Ingredients

1 cup uncooked quinoa
1 large carrot
½ -1 beet
10 cherry tomatoes
1 cup parsley
1-2 stalks celery
1 green onion
½ cup – 1 cup cooked and cooled tempeh (page 188)

Dressing ingredients

½ cup apple cider vinegar or balsamic
2 tbsp. extra virgin olive oil
½ lemon (freshly squeezed)
A few pinches of sea salt

Instructions

Quinoa

- Rinse quinoa and strain
- Bring 2 cups water to a boil and add 1 cup quinoa
- Bring back to a boil, then cover, and cook over medium heat for 12 minutes (until quinoa has absorbed all of the water) – mix occasionally
- Remove from heat, fluff, cover and let stand for 15 minutes
- Place quinoa into a bowl and let it cool, uncovered, for 30 minutes – fluff occasionally

Veggies

- Peel carrot and beet
- Add carrot and parsley to mini blender and blend until chopped
- Cut beet into small bite size pieces
- Chop celery and green onion
- Cut tomatoes into halves or leave whole

Dressing

- Add all dressing ingredients to a small bowl and mix together

Putting it all together

- Add veggies to quinoa
- Add desired amount of tempeh
- Pour dressing on top and enjoy

Apple, Beet and Sweet Potato Quinoa Salad

Ingredients

1 cup uncooked quinoa
1 apple – diced
3 tbsp. currants or unsulphured raisins
½ cup chopped kale
¾ cup cooked sweet potatoes
2 beets - roasted or raw

Dressing ingredients

¼ cup extra virgin olive oil or flaxseed oil
½ fresh lemon (freshly squeezed)
few pinches of sea salt
black pepper to taste

Instructions

Quinoa

- Rinse quinoa and strain
- Bring 2 cups water to a boil and add 1 cup quinoa
- Bring back to a boil, then cover, and cook over medium heat for 12 minutes (until quinoa has absorbed all of the water) – mix occasionally
- Remove from heat, fluff, cover and let stand for 15 minutes
- Place quinoa into a bowl and let it cool, uncovered, for 30 minutes – fluff occasionally

Beets

<u>Roasted beets:</u>

- Place 2 medium size beets (with skin on) in a glass baking dish and drizzle with grape seed or olive oil and a pinch of sea salt
- Bake at 375°F in the oven, uncovered for 45 minutes – 1 hour
- When they begin to soften, remove from oven and let them cool
- Peel off skin and cut into chunks

<u>Raw beets:</u>

- Peel beets using a knife or vegetable peeler
- Cut into chunks

Sweet Potatoes

- Peel a medium sized sweet potato
- Cut into chunks
- Place potatoes in boiling water on the stove or steam them
- Allow to cool
- Can also roast the potatoes in the same baking dish as the beets with a little bit of olive oil and a pinch of sea salt. Bake for 30-45 minutes until soft.

<u>**Putting It All Together**</u>

- Chop kale and dice apple
- Place quinoa into large bowl
- Add beets, sweet potatoes, kale, apple and currants to quinoa
- Combine dressing ingredients in separate bowl and pour on top of quinoa salad
- Serve cold or hot

Sweet Potato Salad

Ingredients

2 medium sweet potatoes - peeled and cubed
¼ cup dried cranberries or raisins
1 medium red onion – cut into small pieces
handful chopped parsley
1 tbsp. olive oil
pinch sea salt and ground pepper

Dressing

2 tbsp. olive oil
2 tsp. Dijon mustard
1 tsp. raw honey or pure maple syrup
¼ tsp. sea salt
pinch of black pepper

Instructions

- Preheat oven to 400°F
- Place potatoes and onions in bowl with olive oil, salt and pepper
- Place onto baking sheet linked with parchment paper and roast at 400 degrees for 30 minutes – until tender
- Prepare dressing: combine all ingredients into small bowl
- Once potatoes are roasted, remove from oven and top with cranberries/raisins
- Add dressing and parsley
- Allow potatoes to cool, place in fridge and serve cold, or serve hot immediately

Whole Grain Pasta Salad

* This pasta salad can be made using a variety of different homemade dressings (listed below) and can be consumed hot or cold.

Ingredients

3-4 cups cooked brown rice pasta, buckwheat pasta, spelt pasta or other whole grain pasta of choice (penne or fusilli work well).
1 red pepper – diced
½ cup sliced carrots
½ cup chopped green onion
½ cup cherry tomatoes – cut in half
* Can use any vegetables you like

Instructions

- Cook pasta and allow to cool
- Cut vegetables and add to pasta
- Prepare your dressing of choice (see recipes below) and pour overtop of pasta

Salad Dressings

Oil and Vinegar Dressing

¼ cup olive oil or flaxseed oil
2-3 tbsp. apple cider vinegar (raw, unpasteurized)
½ fresh squeezed lemon
pinch of sea salt and pepper to taste
* Mix all ingredients together in bowl

Basil Pesto Dressing

3 cups fresh basil
½ cup raw & shelled sunflower seeds or pine nuts (or a combination)
2-3 cloves fresh garlic
¼ cup extra virgin olive oil
½ tsp. sea salt, to taste
* Place all ingredients in food processor and process until smooth

Creamy Avocado Dressing

½ ripe avocado
½ cup plain Greek yogurt
¾ cup fresh cilantro or parsley
1 green onion - chopped
1 clove garlic
1 tbsp. fresh lime juice
½ tsp. sea salt
1 tsp. honey
* Place all ingredients in food processor and process until smooth

Edamame and Avocado Salad

Ingredients

3 cups shelled edamame – cooked
1 avocado chunked
1 green onion chopped
¼ cup chopped parsley
¼ cup kale chopped

Dressing

1 tbsp. olive oil
2 tbsp. apple cider vinegar
1 clove crushed garlic (remove after a few seconds)
grated ginger
pinch of salt and pepper
1 lime

Instructions

- Boil uncooked edamame for 4-5 minutes on medium/high heat
- Strain excess liquid, rinse edamame in cold water and place in the fridge to cool
- Cut avocado into chunks
- Chop green onion
- Chop parsley and kale
- Combine all ingredients into a medium size bowl
- Combine all dressing ingredients in a separate bowl and pour over salad
- Serve cold

SOUPS

Butternut Squash Soup

Ingredients

1 large butternut squash (peeled, seeded and cubed)
¾ of medium onion – diced
2 cloves of garlic – minced
2 stalks celery - chopped
2 large carrots - chopped
2 tbsp. extra virgin olive oil
2 tsp. sea salt (to taste)
1/2 tsp. black pepper to taste
4 cups water (enough to cover the squash in the pot)

Instructions

- In a medium saucepan, add olive oil, onion and garlic and sauté for about 3 minutes on medium/low temp
- Add butternut squash, carrots, celery and water
- Cover and bring to a boil
- Turn heat down and simmer for about 30 minutes, or until butternut squash is soft
- Remove from heat. Use a slotted spoon to scoop out the vegetables and place into food processor. Leaving liquid in the pot
- Process ingredients until smooth. Add back small amount of water and process again. Continue this until desired consistency
- Pour soup back into pot and place on the stove to simmer
- Add salt and pepper to taste
- Serve hot and topped with pumpkin seeds

Split Pea Soup

Ingredients

1 onion - chopped
1 tbsp. olive oil
3-4 cloves garlic – minced
7 ½ cups water
2 cups green split peas
1 cup lima beans
1 ½ tsp. salt
3 carrots – chopped
3 stalks celery – chopped
2 turnips - chopped
½ cup chopped parsley
½ tsp. dried basil
½ tsp. dried thyme
½ tsp. back pepper

Total time: About 2 hours

Instructions

- Add chopped onion, olive oil and garlic to pot and simmer for 3 minutes
- Add water, peas, lima beans and salt
- Cover, bring to a boil and then reduce to low/medium heat
- Add carrots, celery, turnips, parsley and spices and continue to simmer for 2 hours or until tender
- Using a hand blender or potato masher, puree the soup until thick
- Simmer for another 20-30 minutes and serve hot

Broccoli and Cauliflower Soup

Ingredients

1 head of broccoli
1 head of cauliflower
1 medium sweet potato
4 cloves of garlic
1 medium onion
3 tablespoons extra virgin olive oil
7 cups water or vegetable broth
sea salt and pepper to taste

Instructions

- Chop broccoli, cauliflower and potato
- Chop onion and garlic
- In a large soup pot, add the olive oil, chopped onion and chopped garlic and sauté for about 3 minutes until translucent
- Add broccoli, cauliflower and potato to the pot
- Add water or vegetable broth
- Bring to a boil, then reduce to medium heat and cover
- Cook for 15-20 minutes (until vegetables are tender)
- Remove pot from heat, and using a hand blender, blend until it becomes creamy. If you do not have a hand blender you can transfer the contents of the pot into a food processor or blender
- Add sea salt and pepper to taste
- Serve hot
- Allow remaining soup to cool and place in an airtight container in the refrigerator for up to 4 days. Can also freeze leftovers and re-heat on the stove top as needed

CRACKERS, SNACKS & DESSERTS

Scrumptious Honey Sesame Crackers

Ingredients

1.5 cups brown rice flour
2 tbsp. honey
½ tsp. sea salt
½ cup sesame seeds
1/3 cup ground flax seeds
1/3 cup sunflower seeds
1 cup water
2 tbsp. grape seed oil

Topping

1 tbsp. honey

Sea salt (to sprinkle once baked)

Instructions

- Preheat oven to 350°F
- Line rimmed cookie sheet with parchment paper
- Combine all ingredients except water in a bowl
- Add ¾ cups water and stir dough with wooden spoon
- Knead dough with hands until all ingredients are combined (let dough rest for 3 minutes)
- Place dough on baking sheet, and flatten using your hands
- Place a piece of parchment paper on top of dough, and using your hands or a rolling pin, roll out the dough. The thinner the dough, the crispier the crackers
- Using a pizza cutter or knife, score the dough, outlining small squares or rectangles
- Bake for about 10-15 minutes

- Separate the crackers from each other, flip them over one at a time, and continue to bake until deep golden brown (about 10-15 minutes)
- Remove from oven, and using a basting brush, paint the honey over top of the crackers and sprinkle with sea salt
- Place back into the oven for 2-3 minutes
- Cool completely before storing in an airtight container

Chocolate/Avocado Pudding

Ingredients

1.5 avocados
1 banana
¼ cup pure maple syrup
2 tbsp. raw cacao powder or cocoa powder
1 tsp. pure vanilla extract
¼ cup of rice milk or almond milk
Fresh fruit for dipping

Instructions

- Combine all ingredients (except for rice milk) into blender
- Blend until smooth
- Add small amounts of rice milk at a time, until desired consistency
- Place pudding into a bowl and refrigerate for 30 minutes or longer
- Enjoy with fresh fruit

Date Squares – Makes approx. 12 squares

Ingredients
- 2 cups chopped, pitted dates
- ½ cup water
- ½ cup butter or coconut oil
- 1 ¾ cups brown rice flour
- ½ cup sucanat
- ½ tsp. baking soda
- 1 cup rolled oats
- ¼ tsp. sea salt

Instructions
- Preheat oven to 350° F
- Combine dates and water in saucepan and cook, covered, on low for 5-7 minutes, stirring occasionally
- Remove from heat and set aside to cool
- In a large bowl, combine butter and sucanat
- Add flour, baking soda and salt and combine until it is the consistency of dough (can use your hands)
- Add oats and mix with hands
- Grease a 9x9 square baking pan with grape seed oil and place ½ of the dough mixture into the pan, pressing down to form a base
- Add date mixture and spread evenly on top of dough
- Add the second ½ of the dough mixture on top, pressing down evenly
- Bake for 30 minutes
- Allow it to cool completely in pan, then, cut into squares

Chocolate Squash Brownies

Ingredients
- 1 medium squash pureed
- 5 oz. unsweetened chocolate
- ½ cup coconut or grape seed oil
- 4 large eggs (or chia gel equivalent – see page 75)
- 1 ¼ cup sucanat
- 1 ½ tsp. pure vanilla extract
- ½ tsp. sea salt
- 1 ¼ cup brown rice flour
- ¾ tsp. baking powder

Instructions
- Preheat oven to 350° F
- Use a double boiler (a pot with water and a stainless steel bowl on top) to melt the chocolate and butter – place the chocolate and butter into the double boiler and allow it to melt over medium/high heat. Make sure to keep an eye on it so it does not burn
- In a large bowl, beat eggs, sucanat, vanilla and sea salt until combined
- Add melted chocolate to the mixture
- Add pureed squash to the mixture
- Add flour and baking powder to the mixture and whisk/mix until it forms a batter
- Line a muffin tin with paper liners and fill each cup ¾ of the way full
- Bake at 350°F for 15 minutes
- Allow cupcakes to cool completely
- Once cooled, frost the cupcakes with sunflower seed butter or other nut/seed butter and some shredded coconut

Chewy Chocolate Granola Bars

Ingredients

1 cup honey
2/3 cup natural sunflower seed butter (or other nut/seed butter)
2 2/3 cup rolled oats
¾ cup brown rice flour
1 tsp. cinnamon
1.5 cups carob chips (can use dark chocolate chips)
¼ cup ground pumpkin seeds
¼ cup sesame seeds

Instructions

- Combine honey and sunflower seed butter in mixing bowl
- Add in oats, flour, cinnamon, pumpkin seeds and sesame seeds and mix together
- Stir in carob chips
- Lightly grease a 9 x 13 pan with a small amount of coconut oil or grape seed oil
- Press mixture down firmly into pan
- Bake at 350°F for about 12-15 minutes – edges will begin to brown
- Remove from oven and cut into bars or squares, leaving them in the pan after cutting
- Allow bars to cool completely
- Remove bars from pan and enjoy

* Store in an airtight container

Zucchini Banana Loaf – includes option for nut-free

Ingredients

2 cups brown rice flour (or spelt, buckwheat, chickpea flours)
1 tsp. baking powder
½ tsp. baking soda
½ tsp. sea salt
3 ripe bananas – mashed
¼ cup grated zucchini
2 eggs (or chia gel equivalent – see page 75)
1 tsp. ground cinnamon
½ cup coconut sugar or sucanat
1 tbsp. pure maple syrup
½ cup almond milk (or other milk alternative)
¼ cup chopped nuts (almonds, walnuts, pecans, etc.)
handful raw, whole pumpkin seeds – to top with

- *For nut-free version, use brown rice or hemp milk, as well as a combination of seeds instead of chopped nuts (pumpkin seeds, flax seeds, sesame seeds).*

Instructions

- Combine flour, baking powder, baking soda, cinnamon and sea salt in a bowl
- In a separate bowl, combine bananas, eggs, sugar, maple syrup, zucchini and almond milk
- Mix wet and dry ingredients together in a large bowl
- Add in nuts or seeds
- Grease a 4 x 8 inch loaf pan with grape seed oil and pour mixture into pan.
- Top with raw, whole pumpkin seeds
- Bake for 45 minutes – 1 hour at 350°F
- Allow zucchini banana loaf to cool before removing from pan and serving

The Gunk-Free Diet Grocery List

The following list is comprised of healthy, nourishing foods. In fact, this list contains foods that should be present in every healthy kitchen.

You do NOT need to purchase every item on this list. It is simply a guideline to give you a better idea of what to look for when grocery shopping. As you go through this book, you will begin to formulate your own grocery list based on these healthy foods, and will quickly learn which foods you want to consume more of and which ones you do not.

There are some brand names listed as well for many of these items. Again, these are just suggestions. You do NOT have to purchase the recommended brands, and in fact, it is a good idea for you to read product labels while grocery shopping and choose brands that suit you best.

For information on how to read products labels see page 2.

The "Gunk-Free Diet" Grocery List

Protein

Protein powder

- ☐ **Sunwarrior, Vega One or Genuine Health** vegan protein
- ☐ Other vegan protein (no additives or artificial/refined sweeteners)
- ☐ Other 100% New Zealand whey protein isolate/concentrate (no additives or artificial/refined sweeteners)

Legumes - *Purchase raw beans to be cooked or canned beans (Eden Organic - low in sodium and in BPA free cans)*

- ☐ Chickpeas
- ☐ Kidney Beans
- ☐ Lentils
- ☐ Navy beans
- ☐ Peas
- ☐ Pinto beans
- ☐ Red lentils
- ☐ Black Beans
- ☐ Adzuki beans
- ☐ Mixed beans
- ☐ Split peas
- ☐ Mung beans
- ☐ Soybeans (edamame) – frozen
- ☐ Tofu (sprouted)
- ☐ Tempeh – **Noble Bean**

Fish – *wild caught when possible*

- ☐ Salmon
- ☐ Mackerel
- ☐ Halibut

- ☐ Tuna
- ☐ Cod
- ☐ Haddock
- ☐ Sardines
- ☐ Snapper
- ☐ Tuna
- ☐ Trout
- ☐ Tilapia

Poultry – *lean, free-range & organic when possible*
- ☐ Chicken (fresh or ground – not processed)
- ☐ Turkey (fresh or ground - not processed)
- ☐ Quail
- ☐ Duck

Red Meat – *lean, grass-fed & organic when possible (consume red meat in moderation).*
- ☐ Beef
- ☐ Lamb
- ☐ Venison
- ☐ Veal

Eggs - *free-run*

Nuts and seeds - *raw, unsalted* – *Navitas Naturals, PRANA, Bob's Red Mill*
- ☐ Almonds
- ☐ Cashews
- ☐ Brazil nuts
- ☐ Walnuts

- ☐ Macadamia nuts
- ☐ Pecans
- ☐ Sesame seeds
- ☐ Sunflower seeds
- ☐ Pumpkin seeds
- ☐ Flax seeds
- ☐ Hemp seeds – **Manitoba Harvest**
- ☐ Chia seeds

Nut and seed butters - *organic when possible, free of refined sugar*
- ☐ Nut butters - **Nuts To You**
- ☐ Sunflower seed butter – **Sunbutter**
- ☐ Pumpkin seed butter – **Omega Nutrition**
- ☐ Tahini
- ☐ Organic peanut butter (avoid non-organic peanut butter)

Carbohydrates

Breads – *Stonemill, Ezekiel, Manna, Udi's Gluten-Free*
- ☐ 100% whole grain (for those with gluten sensitivities, avoid rye, spelt, wheat, and oats)

Cereals

Nature's Path, Enjoy Life, Bob's Red Mill, Dorset Cereals, Barbara's Bakery

Hot Cereals
- ☐ Oatmeal (plain steel cut oats or rolled oats) – avoid instant oatmeal with added flavors/sugar. Opt for gluten-free oats when possible.
- ☐ Quinoa and/or quinoa flakes (raw grains to be cooked)
- ☐ Oat bran

Dry Cereals

☐ 100% whole grain cereal without added sugar

☐ Quinoa puffs

☐ Brown rice cereal

☐ Granola (without added sugar)

Whole grains/Pasta/Rice/Flour

☐ Quinoa

☐ Buckwheat

☐ Spelt

☐ Rye

☐ Brown rice and brown rice pasta

☐ 100% whole wheat

☐ Millet

☐ Barley

☐ Kamut

☐ Corn

☐ Teff

☐ Amaranth

Crackers – Mary's Gone Crackers, Late July, Glutino, Enerjive

☐ Brown rice crackers

☐ 100% whole grain crackers

☐ Plain rice cakes

Cookies/Snacks

Sweets From the Earth, Oskri, Enerjive, Mary's Gone Crackers, Udi's Gluten Free, Enjoy Life, Giddy Yoyo, Nud Fud, Annie's, Late July, GoGo Quinoa

☐ Cookies and snacks made with whole grains, no added sugar, color or artificial ingredients.

Fruits & Vegetables

Any and all fruits and vegetables are acceptable, except those that cause a reaction. Avoid grapefruit if on medication.

Vegetables – *organic when possible*
- ☐ Collard greens
- ☐ Kale
- ☐ Spinach
- ☐ Broccoli
- ☐ Cauliflower
- ☐ Bok choy
- ☐ Carrots
- ☐ Celery
- ☐ Beets
- ☐ Tomato
- ☐ Cucumber
- ☐ Bell peppers
- ☐ Eggplant
- ☐ Mushrooms
- ☐ Sweet potato
- ☐ Butternut squash
- ☐ Asparagus
- ☐ Zucchini
- ☐ Other fresh vegetables
- ☐ Frozen vegetables – **Cookin' Greens**

Fruits – *organic when possible*
- ☐ Avocado
- ☐ Blueberries
- ☐ Blackberries

- ☐ Raspberries
- ☐ Strawberries
- ☐ Oranges
- ☐ Lemons
- ☐ Apples
- ☐ Pears
- ☐ Bananas
- ☐ Grapes
- ☐ Cherries
- ☐ Kiwi fruit
- ☐ Watermelon
- ☐ Limes
- ☐ Pomegranate

Frozen fruit

- ☐ Blueberries
- ☐ Raspberries
- ☐ Strawberries
- ☐ Mango

Dairy and Dairy Alternatives

Dairy (organic when possible)

- ☐ Goat cheese
- ☐ Sheep cheese
- ☐ Plain, unsweetened or naturally sweetened Greek Yogurt
- ☐ Kefir

Dairy Alternatives

- ☐ Rice milk - **Ryza, Rice Dream**
- ☐ Almond milk - **Almond Breeze, Silk True Almond**

- ☐ Hemp milk - **Manitoba Harvest Hemp Bliss**
- ☐ Coconut milk
- ☐ Organic or fermented soymilk
- ☐ Organic or fermented soy or coconut yogurt – **Yoso**
- ☐ Vegan cheese – **Daiya**

Good Fats/Oils – unrefined, cold-pressed oils

- ☐ Organic butter or Ghee (clarified butter)
- ☐ Coconut oil
- ☐ High oleic sunflower oil
- ☐ Sesame seed oil
- ☐ Extra-virgin olive oil
- ☐ Avocado oil
- ☐ Grape seed oil
- ☐ Flax seed oil – **Omega Nutrition**
- ☐ Hemp seed oil - **Manitoba Harvest**

Vinegars/Sauces/Dressings

- ☐ Unpasteurized apple cider vinegar – **Braggs**
- ☐ Organic balsamic vinegar
- ☐ Rice vinegar
- ☐ Red wine vinegar
- ☐ Wheat-free soy sauce – **San-J Tamari, Braggs**
- ☐ Salad dressings without MSG or added sugar – **RawFoodz, Annie's**

Flours – Bob's Red Mill, Oak Manor

- ☐ Brown rice flour
- ☐ Quinoa flour
- ☐ Buckwheat flour
- ☐ Whole-wheat flour

- ☐ Millet flour
- ☐ Oat flour
- ☐ Coconut flour
- ☐ Chickpea flour

Sweeteners
- ☐ Raw or Manuka honey - **NudeBee, Wedderspoon**
- ☐ Pure maple syrup
- ☐ Stevia (liquid or powder)
- ☐ Sucanat
- ☐ Molasses
- ☐ Cane juice
- ☐ Coconut sugar – **Organika**
- ☐ Brown rice syrup

Spices/Herbs/Seaweeds – Spice Sanctuary
- ☐ Basil
- ☐ Bay leaves
- ☐ Rosemary
- ☐ Tumeric
- ☐ Chili Pepper
- ☐ Coriander
- ☐ Fenugreek
- ☐ Chives
- ☐ Black Pepper
- ☐ Cardamom
- ☐ Cayenne
- ☐ Nutmeg
- ☐ Oregano
- ☐ Parsley (fresh)
- ☐ Cinnamon

- ☐ Cloves
- ☐ Black pepper
- ☐ Cumin
- ☐ Sea salt
- ☐ Thyme
- ☐ Dill (fresh)
- ☐ Fennel Seeds
- ☐ Garlic (fresh and/or powder)
- ☐ Ginger (fresh and/or powder)
- ☐ Mustard Seeds

Seaweeds
- ☐ Kelp
- ☐ Kombu
- ☐ Arame
- ☐ Wakame
- ☐ Nori

Other/Superfoods/Supplements Baking Powder
- ☐ Baking Soda
- ☐ Carob powder
- ☐ Raw cocoa powder
- ☐ Xantham gum
- ☐ Applesauce (unsweetened)
- ☐ Cocoa nibs or powder
- ☐ Sauerkraut (fermented)
- ☐ Sea salt
- ☐ Pure vanilla extract
- ☐ Vegetable or chicken stock
- ☐ Nutritional yeast

- ☐ Mustard
- ☐ Gogi berries – **Prana, Navitas Naturals**
- ☐ Spirulina powder
- ☐ Matcha green tea powder – **DO matcha**
- ☐ Wheatgrass - **Amazing Grass**
- ☐ Aloe juice or gel – **Lily of the Desert**
- ☐ Probiotics – **Udo's**
- ☐ Fish oil - **Ascenta Health**
- ☐ Magnesium Powder – **Natural Calm**
- ☐ Dried unsweetened coconut
- ☐ Grape skin powder – **Bioflavia**

Dried Fruit – PRANA, Navitas Naturals
- ☐ Dates
- ☐ Prunes
- ☐ Figs
- ☐ Dried cranberries
- ☐ Currants
- ☐ Unsulphured raisins

All dried fruit should be unsweetened, without sulfites

Beverages and Herbal Teas (loose leaf tea)
- ☐ Ginger tea
- ☐ Rooibos tea
- ☐ Chamomile tea
- ☐ Dandelion tea
- ☐ Peppermint tea
- ☐ Lavender tea
- ☐ Licorice tea
- ☐ Coconut water – **Coco the Drink**

Natural Beauty Care and Cleaning Products

- ☐ Green Beaver
- ☐ Pangea organics
- ☐ Natracare
- ☐ Pure+Simple
- ☐ Badger
- ☐ Dr.Bronner
- ☐ Ecover

Acknowledgements

This book was written for you – you, who picked it up and decided that you were going to allow it to be a part of your life. Without you, there would be no book, and my ultimate goal of sharing this information with those who need it would never have been possible. So, thank you.

I literally would not be where I am today without the love, support and encouragement from my family. Coming from a family of four kids, and having the most amazing mother on the planet, I have always been so fortunate to have such a great support group. I am the person that I am today because of my sister Alison, my brothers Jordan and Evan, and my mom Rhonda.

I feel so lucky to have been blessed with such an amazing family-in-law. Mark, Brenda, Ben, Alana and Daniel, thank you all for your constant support and encouragement.

Emily and Deanna, my trusted team, who worked diligently (and patiently) with me as the final pages of this book came together. Thank you for being my sounding board, for your honest input, and for all of your help in making this book come to life. I am so lucky to have such dedicated and passionate people to work with everyday. Go team!

My husband (and biggest fan), Jarryd, has made so much of this possible for me. Truly, without him, I would have never had the courage to go back to school to study nutrition, and would never have made the amazing changes in my life that led to the writing of this book. It was with his encouragement and daily support (he would literally spend hours reading and re-reading with me) that I finally had the opportunity to live my dream of doing what I knew I was born to do. His patience and understanding while writing this book deserves an award. The long nights, early mornings, and frequent calls to edit and give his advice over and over again, is something that I will always be grateful for. He was my prized guinea pig, who was always first in line to taste the recipes created for this book. The mere look on his face would decide whether or not the recipes were a "yay" or "nay". Thanks Jar, for everything you do for me everyday and for your patience and dedication to this book.

Resources

Enerjive
Nutrient packed gluten-free, quinoa skinny crackers
Enerjive Inc.
59 Iber Road.
Stittsville, ON K2S 1E7
613.829.9094
www.enerjivefood.com

Yoso
Dairy-free and gluten-free yogurts and spreads
Cambridge, Ontario
(866) 887-YOSO (9676)
www.yoso.ca

Manitoba Harvest
High quality hemp foods and oils
69 Eagle Drive
Winnipeg, Manitoba
R2R 1V4
204-953-0233
1-800-665-HEMP(4367)
www.manitobaharvest.com

Prana
Organic & vegan products; nuts, dried fruits, seeds, sweet & savoury snacks, trail mix, superfoods, cacao and coconut products
160 Saint-Viateur E, suite #500
Montreal, Quebec
H2T 1A8
514 276-4864
www.pranana.com

Coco the Drink
Natural coconut water beverage
www.cocothenaturaldrink.com

Ascenta Health
High quality fish oil supplements
Ascenta Health Ltd.
4-15 Garland Avenue
Dartmouth, NS
B3B 0A6
902.435.7329
Toll Free: 866.224.1775
www.ascentahealth.com

Enjoy Life Foods
Gluten-free and allergy friendly snack foods; cookies, bars, fruit mixes, chocolates & cereals
www.enjoylifefoods.com

Wedderspoon
Organic bee products
1-888-256-6603
www.wedderspoon.ca

Sunbutter
Natural sunflower seed spreads
Red River Commodities 501 42nd St. NW
Fargo, ND 58102
1-800-437-5539
www.sunbutter.com

RawFoodz
Raw, nutrient-rich dressings
416-720-3151 (Sher Kopman)
416-995-4021 (Michelle Cass)
www.rawfoodz.ca

Narural Calm
Highly absorbable magnesium and calcium products
5 Idleswift Dr.
Thornhill, Ontario, L4J 1K6
(905)-762-8910 or (866)-854-2256
www.naturalcalm.ca

Spice Sanctuary
High quality, premium spices
Canmore, Alberta
403 389 3743
www.spicesanctuary.com

NudFud
Raw, organic, gluten-free snacks
11 Carlaw Avenue
Toronto, Ontario
M4M 2R6
647-351-9000
www.nudfud.com

Sweets From the Earth
Natural vegan snacks and desserts
43 Mulock Ave
Toronto, Ontario
M6N 3C3
647-436-2004
888-886-2004
www.sweetsfromtheearth.com

Naturally Savvy
Resource for natural & organic living
www.naturallysavvy.com

Mind Body Green
Wellness guide
www.mindbodygreen.com

Natural News
Health and wellness news
www.naturalnews.com

Selected References

Alexander, D., Manier, J., and Callahan, P. "For Every Fad, Another Cookie: How Science and Diet Crazes Confuse Consumers, Reshape Recipes and Fail, Ultimately, to Reform Eating Habits." *Chicago Tribune*, August 23, 2005.

American Heart Association [AHA]. 2005. "The No Fad Diet: A Personal Plan For Healthy Weight Loss." New York: Clarkson Potter.

American Heart Association. "Make Healthy Food Choices." April 4, 2008. www.americanheart.org/presenter.jhtml?identifier=537

Arrieta, M.C., et al. 2006. *Gut.* 55(10): 1512-1520.

Associated Press: "Irregular Sleep Tied to Obesity, Other Health Problems." *USA Today*, May 7, 2008. www.usatoday.com/news/health/2008-05-07-sleep-obesity_N.htm

Balch, J.F. Prescription for Natural Cures. New Jersey: John Wiley and Sons, Inc, 2004.

Bateson-Koch, C. 1994. *Allergies: Disease in Disguise*. Alive Books. Burnaby BC.

Brownell, K.D., and K.B. Horgen. 2004. Food Fight: *The Inside Story of the Food Industry, America's Obesity Crisis, and what we can do about it.* New York: McGraw-Hill.

Burstain, T. "Balancing Your Hunger Hormones." www.hungerhormones.com (accessed November 6, 2012.)

Campbell TC. "The Dietary causes of degenerative diseases: nutrients vs. foods." In: N.J. Temple and D.P. Burkitt (eds.) Western Diseases: their dietary prevention and reversibility, pp. 119-152. Totowa, NJ: Human Press, 1994.

Centre for Science in the Public Interest. "Chemical Cuisine: A Guide to Food Additives." *Nutrition Action Health Letter*, May 2008.

Colbin, A. 1996. Food and Healing. Ballantine Books. NY, NY. Dodd, R., BSC, ND. Pers. Comm. www.naturalpath-cancerclinic.com. Mississauga, ON.

Collins, K. "Fight Cancer with Dark Green Vegetables: Average Adult Should Eat Three Cups of Produce a Week." MSNBC.com, April 8,2005. http://www.msnbc.com/id/7421199/

Cummings, L C. 1986. "The Political Reality of Artificial Sweeteners." In Sapolsky, ed., 1986, 116-40.

Dixon, S. "Food for Thought: The Facts on Fiber." *Progress Newsletter* (newsletter, University of Michigan Comprehensive Cancer Center, winter 2002) www.cancer.med.umich.edu/news/pro09win02.shtml#four

Dufty, William (1975). *Sugar Blues.* Chilton Book Company, Padnor, PA, USA. Warner Brooks, Inc., NY.

Dunn, A.L., et al. 2005. American Journal of Preventative Medicine. 28(1): 1-8.

Eades, M. "A Spoonful of Sugar," The Blog of Michael R. Eades, M.D., http:// www.proteinpower.com/drmike/ sugar-and-sweeteners/a-spoonful-of-sugar.

Environmental Working Group. http://www.ewg.org/foodnews/

Erasmus, Udo. Fats that Heal. Fats that Kill. Tennessee: Alive Books, 1993.

Field, A., et al. "Association of Weight Change, Weight Control Practices, and Weight Cycling among Women in The Nurse's Health

Study II. *"International Journal of Obesity and Related Metabolic Disorders* 28, no. 9 (September, 2004).

Hill, J.O., and J.C. Peters. 1998. "Environmental Contributions to the Obesity Epidemic."

Fowler, S.P. 65th Annual Scientific Sessions, American Diabetes Association, San Diego, June 10-14, 2005; Abstract 1058-P.

Frusztajer, N.T., and J.J. Wurtman 2009. *The Serotonin Power Diet*. Rodale Press. Emmaus, PA.

Furness, J.B., et al. 1999. *Gastrointestinal and Liver Physiology*. 277 (5): G922-G928.

Gottschall, E.G. 1994. *Breaking The Vicious Cycle*. Kirkton Press, Kirkton, ON.

Graci, S. 2001. *The Food Connection*. MacMillan Canada. Toronto, ON.

Hass, Elson M. Staying Healthy With Nutrition. California: Celestial Arts, 2006.

Inclusion of fish or fish oil in weight-loss diets for young adults: effects on blood lipids. *International Journal of Obesity* (2008) 32, 1105–1112; published online 20 May 2008.

International Food Information Council. "Functional Foods Fact Sheet: Plant Stanols and Sterols." July 2007 www.ific.org/publications/factsheets/sterolfs.cfm.

International Food Information Council. "2012 What's In Our Food: Understanding Common Food Ingredients" August 25, 2012. http://www.ific.org.

International Obesity TaskForce. "Edocrine Disruptors in Common Plastics Linked to Obesity Risk." ScienceDaily, May 15, 2008. www.sciencedaily.com/releases/2008/05/080514091427.htm

Isaacs, S. *The Leptin Boost Diet*. Berkely, CA: Ulysses Press, 2007.

Jump, D.B., et al. 1999. *Prostaglandins, Leukotrines and Essential Fatty Acids*. 60(5-6): 345-349.

Kuzemchak, S. "Outsmart Your Cravings." *Prevention*, February 2008.

Logan, A.C. 2004. *Lipids in Health and Disease*. 3: 25.

Lipka, Mitch. "What do Your Food Labels Really Mean, 'Free Range','Natural','Non-Toxic', and Other Myths"

Liu, S., et al. "A Prospective Study of Whole-Grain Intake and Risk of Type 2 Diabetes Mellitus in US Women." *American Journal of Public Health* 90, no. 9 (2000).

McArdle, W. *Exercise Physiology: Energy, Nutrition and Human Performance*. Philadelphia: Lippincott Williams & Wilkins, April 2006.

Manier,J.,Callaham, P., and Alexander, D. "The Oreo, Obesity and Us: craving the Cookie: The Brain is Wired to Love Sweets, but Are They Addictive? America's Iconic Cookie Captures the Nation's Burgeoning Dietary Dilemma." *Chicago Tribune*, August 21, 2005.

Mann, N. 2000. *European Journal of Nutrition*. 39(2): 71-79.

Mcginnis, W.R., et al. 2008. *Alternative Therapies in Health and Medicine*. 14(2): 40-50.

Meyer, K., et al. "Carbohydrates, Dietary Fibre, and Incident Type 2 Diabetes in Older Women." *American Journal of Clinical Nutrition* 71, no. 4 (2000).

Mozaffarian, D., et al. "Trans Fatty Acids and Cardiovascular Disease." *New England Journal of Medicine* 354, no. 15 (April 13, 2006).

Murray, M.T., and J. Pizzorono. 1998. *Encyclopedia of Natural Medicine*. Revised 2nd ed. Prima Publishing. Rosedale, CA.

National Digestive Diseases Information Clearinghouse (NNDDIC). "Your Digestive System and How It Works." NIH publication no. 08-2681, April 2008.

Nikfar, S., et al. 2008. *Diseases of the Colon and Rectum*. 51(12): 1775-1780.

SELECTED REFERENCES

Park, Alice (2010) Study: "Too Much Sugar Increases Heart Risk." Time Magazine: Health and Family, April 21, 2010. www.time.com/time/health/article/0,8599,1983542,00.html.

Peterson, S., et al. 2006. *Food and Chemical Toxicity*. 44(9): 1474-1484.

Physicians for Social Responsibility. "Environmental Endocrine Disruptors: What Health Care Providers Should Know." www.psr.org/site/DocServer/Environmental_Endocrine_Disruptors.pdf.

Princeton University. "Sugar Can Be Addictive," Physorg.com, December 10, 2010. [November 2, 2012] http:// www.physorg.com/news148116045.html.

Reeds, P.J., and D.G Burrin. 2001. *Journal of Nutrition*. 131 (Suppl.9): 2505S-2508S.

Roizen, M., and Oz, M. *You: On a Diet: The Owner's Manual for Waist Management*. New York: Free Press, 2006.

Sargeant, D. 1999. *Hard to Swallow*. Alive Books. Burnaby BC.

Schmidt, Elaine. Eating more omega-3 fatty acids can offset damage, researchers say. May 15, 2012 http://newsroom.ucla.edu/portal/ucla/this-is-your-brain-on-sugar-ucla-233992.aspx

Sears, B. 2005. The Anti-Inflammation Zone. HarperCollins. NY, NY.

Solan, M. 2009. *Natural Health*. 39(6): 78-79.

Spalding, K., et al. "Dynamics of Fat Cell Turnover in Humans." *Nature* 453, no. 7196 (June 5, 2008).

The Merck Manuals Online Medical Library - http://www.merckmanuals.com

The World's Healthiest Foods - http://www.whfoods.com

Tsimihodimos V, et al. Cola-induced hypokalaemia: pathophysiological mechanisms and clinical implications. *International Journal of Clinical Practice*. 2009; 63: 900-902.

USDA Economic Research Service. "Dietary Assessment of Major Trends in the U.S. Food Consumption, 1970-2005/EIB-33." www.ers.usda.gov/Publications/EIB33/Eib33.pdf (March 2008).

Verdu, E.F., et al. 2007. *Canadian Journal of Gastroenterology.* 21(7): 435-455.

Wang YC, et al. Impact of change in sweetened caloric beverage consumption on energy intake among children and adolescents. *Archives of Pediatric and Adolescent Medicine.* 2009;163:336-343.

Wansink, B. *Mindless Eating.* New York: Bantam Dell, 2006.

Watson, B. 2002. *Renew Your Life.* Renew Life Press. Clearwater, FL.

World's Healthiest Foods http://www.whfoods.com

Zeuzem, S. 2000. *International Journal of Colorectal Diseases.* 15(2): 59-82.

Index

aging (anti), 70, 131
alcohol, 35-36, 156
alkaline/alkalinize, 83, 92, 97, 106-107
allergies, 52, 57, 60-61, 144
antibiotics
  in food, 58, 78
  interactions/effects, 82, 121
antioxidants, 29-32, 54, 69, 81, 83, 101, 106-108, 129
anxiety
  contributing factors, 27-28, 37, 39, 134-135
  relief from, 33, 108, 138
artificial
  color, 2, 4, 20, 41, 43, 78, 90, 114, 118
  flavor, 3, 4, 20, 28, 41, 43, 78, 114, 118
  sweetener, 20, 28, 39, 43, 76, 114
blood sugar, 5, 31, 38, 42, 44-51, 67, 74, 82, 94, 101, 107, 110, 126

blood pressure, 30, 32, 66, 68, 81, 94, 108, 112, 114, 134
bpa-free, 49, 90
breakfast, 5, 10, 47, 92, 96, 117, 159
calcium
  good sources, 32, 41, 46, 59, 61-62, 70, 81, 83, 102, 105, 129
  calcium loss, 27-28, 38, 59
carbohydrates, 6, 17, 38-39, 44-45, 48, 157
carcinogen, 81, 142
cardiovascular health (also heart disease), 31, 33, 39, 45, 58, 66, 68, 71-72, 104-105, 108, 110-111, 113, 128, 134-135
celiac disease, 20, 52
cellulite, 131
chemicals (to avoid), 35, 78, 90, 142-144, 147-148, 163
cholesterol (high), 31-33, 45-46, 48, 50, 66, 68-71, 74-75, 80, 82, 102, 104, 110-111, 112, 122, 127-129

coconut, 18-19, 30, 53, 54, 62-64, 68-70, 110-111, 114, 144-147
coffee, 21, 26-27
  substitutes, 29-33
cravings, 37-39, 44, 48, 74, 89, 96, 101, 107, 110
dairy, 18, 20-21, 57-65, 67, 78, 157
  alternatives, 18, 59-65, 78
detoxification, 31, 35, 50, 81, 83, 88, 92-97, 100-101, 106-107, 109, 112-113, 127-128, 130-131, 159, 160
diabetes (see also, blood sugar)
  foods for, 31, 45-46, 68, 70, 112
  foods to avoid, 37-38, 44, 66-67, 75, 82, 108
digestion,
  ways to improve, 32-33, 36, 52, 77, 83, 88, 92-94, 107, 109, 121, 124, 128, 131
  causes of poor digestion, 133, 135
dinner, 5, 12
dry skin, 70, 131, 144, 146
dry skin brushing, 131, 132, 160
enzymes (in food), 61, 78, 80, 94, 96-97, 107, 124
exercise, 89, 112-113, 159
fat (body fat), 2-4, 6, 35-36, 38, 66, 94, 108
  bad fat (saturated and trans), 2, 4, 20, 58, 66-67, 75, 158
  good fat (also essential fatty acids), 5, 18, 54, 62, 66-69, 72, 102, 104-105, 108, 110-111, 157-158, 218
fatigue, 26, 38, 52, 110, 134, 138
fermented foods, 18, 36, 60-61, 77, 121-124
fiber, 40, 44-51, 54, 80, 83, 101-107, 122-124, 157
flour, 17-18, 20, 45-46, 53-55, 157, 185, 215, 218-219
gluten,
  sensitivity/celiac disease, 17, 20, 52-55, 214
  gluten-free foods, 10-11, 47, 53-55, 103, 214
heartburn, 27, 32,
heart disease
  (see cardiovascular health)
high blood pressure
  (see blood pressure)
hormones, 30, 67, 76, 105, 133-136, 142-143
  in food (synthetic), 58, 75, 78, 90
hydrogenated, 2, 4, 20, 67
immune system
  protect/boost, 32-33, 40, 67, 70, 81, 88, 108-110, 121, 124, 126, 128, 131, 134, 136, 161
  reaction, 52
inflammation
  anti-inflammatory, 31, 32-33, 66-68, 70-73, 80-81, 88, 101-102, 104-105, 107-109, 127-129

causes of inflammation, 21, 52, 57, 67
irritable bowel, 57, 134
legumes, 5-6, 16, 44, 48-49, 51, 74, 158, 212
lemon (benefits), 92-94, 138, 159
liver (detoxification of), 31-32, 35, 36, 81, 92-93, 108, 127
lunch, 5, 11
maca, 26, 29, 30, 156
magnesium
   deficiency, 27, 135
   in food/supplement, 41, 54, 62, 70, 83, 102, 105-106, 135-136, 162-163
matcha, 31, 221
meal planning, 5-13
metabolism, 67, 88, 92-94, 108, 159
monounsaturated (see fat)
osteoporosis, 39, 68, 112
omega-3 fatty acid (see fat)
polyunsaturated (see fat)
probiotics
   in food, 77, 121-124, 160
   supplement, 124, 160
protein
   dietary sources, 16, 47, 51, 54, 74-76, 77, 102, 105-106, 117, 122, 157, 212-213
   powder, 77-78, 118, 212
   daily needs, 5, 74-75, 157
saturated fat (see fat)
seeds
   chia seeds, 51-52, 54, 68, 75, 101-103
   hemp seeds, 52, 62, 68, 72, 105
   flax seeds, 51-52, 54, 68-69, 72-73, 75, 103-105
skin (see dry skin)
sleep
   difficulty sleeping, 6, 36, 134
   sleep aids, 32-33, 134-135, 137, 161-162
soda (pop), 26-28, 156
soy, 76-77, 122-123
spices, 19, 126-130, 160, 219
stress
   negative effects, 133-134, 139
   managing, 30, 32-33, 112, 134-140, 162
sugar (also sweetener)
   negative effects, 3-4, 28, 37-38, 44, 154
   natural sources, 18, 40-43, 157, 215, 219
   sources to avoid, 4, 20, 28, 39, 44, 96, 114
   artificial sweeteners (see artificial)
superfoods, 19, 30, 101-111, 119, 159, 220
supplements, 19, 59, 61, 69, 72, 73, 108, 121, 124, 135-137, 220
trans fat (see fat)
water, 88-90, 159

weight management, 3, 28, 31-32, 36-37, 45, 50, 52, 66-72, 77, 89, 94, 96-97, 101, 107-108, 111-112, 126, 129-130

whole grains, 6, 17, 44-55, 157, 214-215

yoga, 137

About the Author

Shannon Kadlovski, BA, CNP, is a Certified Nutritionist and Healthy Lifestyle Specialist. She is a well sought-after public speaker, and leads a variety of corporate wellness programs, workshops and hands-on classes. She is a freelance writer and has written health and wellness articles for a variety of magazines including, the Huffington Post, Tonic, and Naturally Savvy. She is also the nutrition expert and community producer for "Healthy Helpings" on Rogers TV. Shannon is a faculty member at the Institute of Holistic Nutrition, where she teaches "Holistic Food Preparation".

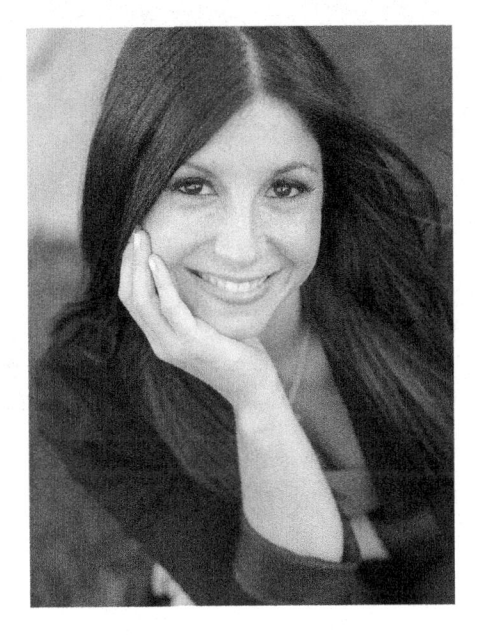

Shannon is the creator and coach of **"Get the Gunk Out – The 21-Day Healthy Living Jump-Start Program"** - a virtual, interactive wellness program available at www.shannonkadlovski.com

Shannon is also the founder of the **"Gunk-Free Project"**, a worldwide revolution dedicated to making healthy living simple and accessible for all. Her mission is to provide free resources and free community events that educate and inspire others to live gunk-free. For information on how to participate in "Gunk-Free Fridays", how to take advantage of tons of free resources, as well as how to start a "Gunk-Free Group" in your area, visit www.shannonkadlovski.com/gunkfreeproject.

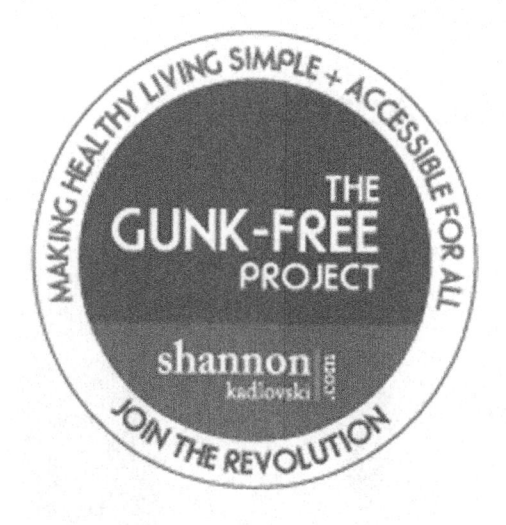

Shannon's approach to health is simple – eat wholesome, natural, clean foods as much as possible and try to minimize the amount of processing and chemicals involved. Don't give up the foods you love, just choose healthier versions of them. Don't take yourself too seriously or be too hard on yourself, it's all about balance.

JOIN SHANNON'S COMMUNITY AND CONNECT WITH THOUSANDS OF OTHERS WHO ARE LIVING GUNK-FREE AT www.shannonkadlovski.com

Made in the USA
Monee, IL
04 May 2021